BYUNG-HI &
BYUNG-SOON LIM

—

KIMCHI

ESSENTIAL RECIPES
OF THE
KOREAN KITCHEN

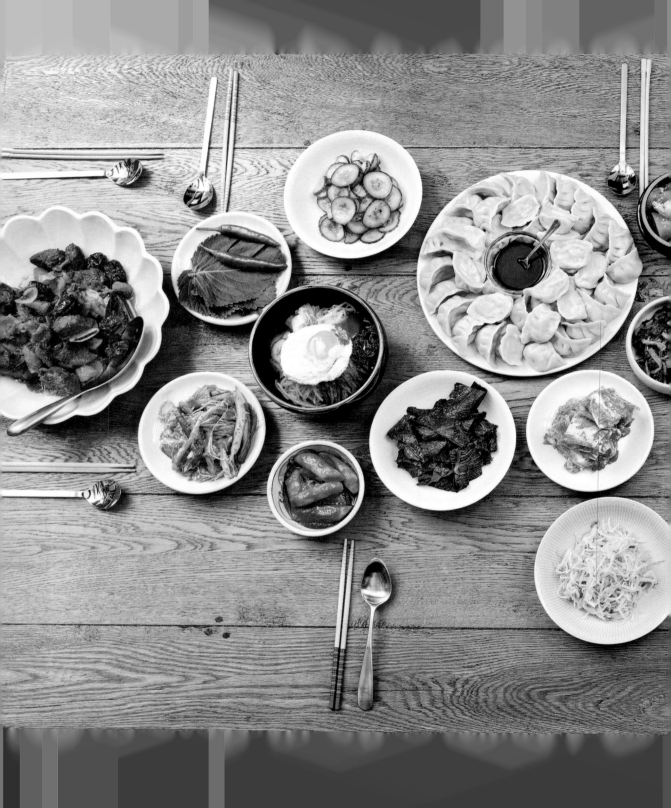

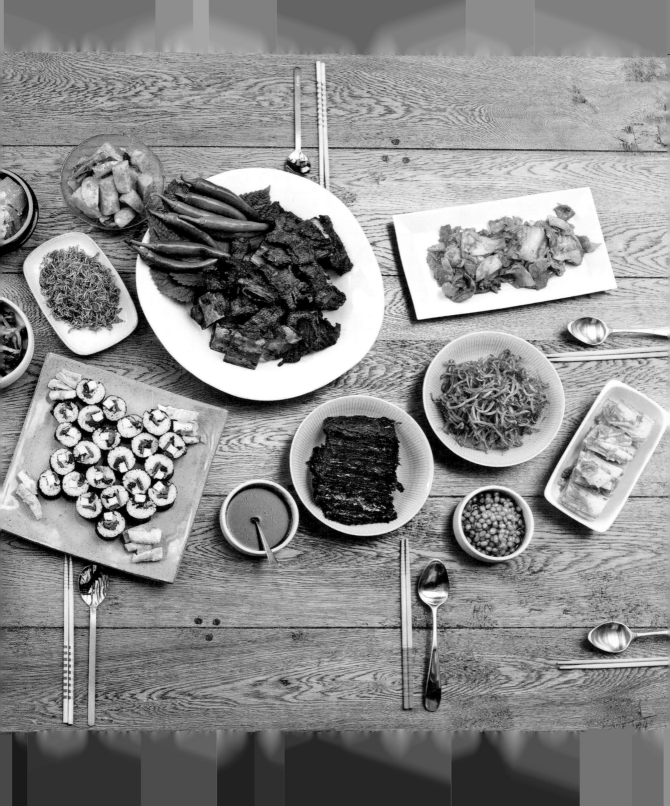

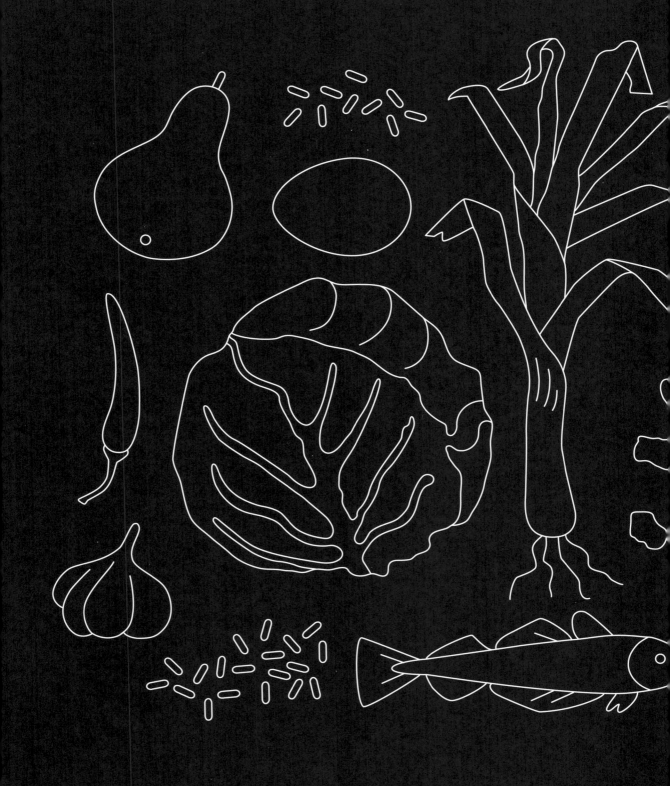

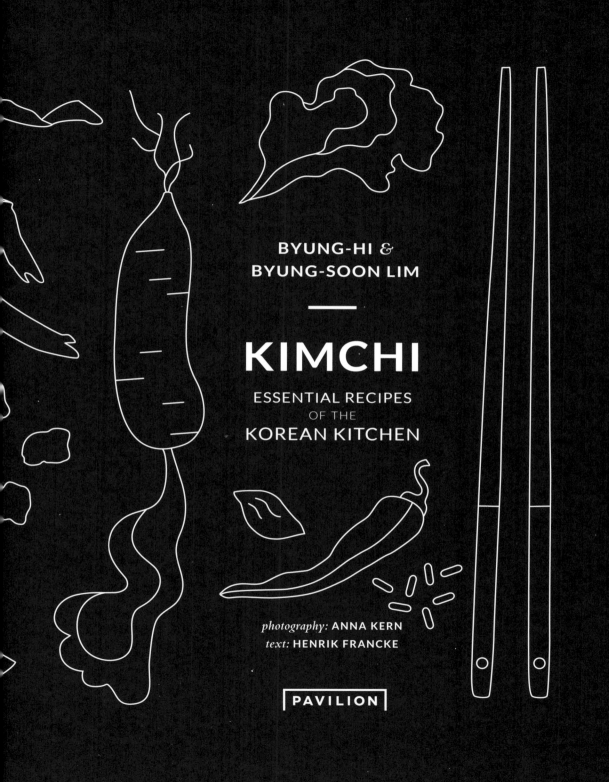

BYUNG-HI &
BYUNG-SOON LIM

—

KIMCHI

ESSENTIAL RECIPES
OF THE
KOREAN KITCHEN

photography: ANNA KERN
text: HENRIK FRANCKE

PAVILION

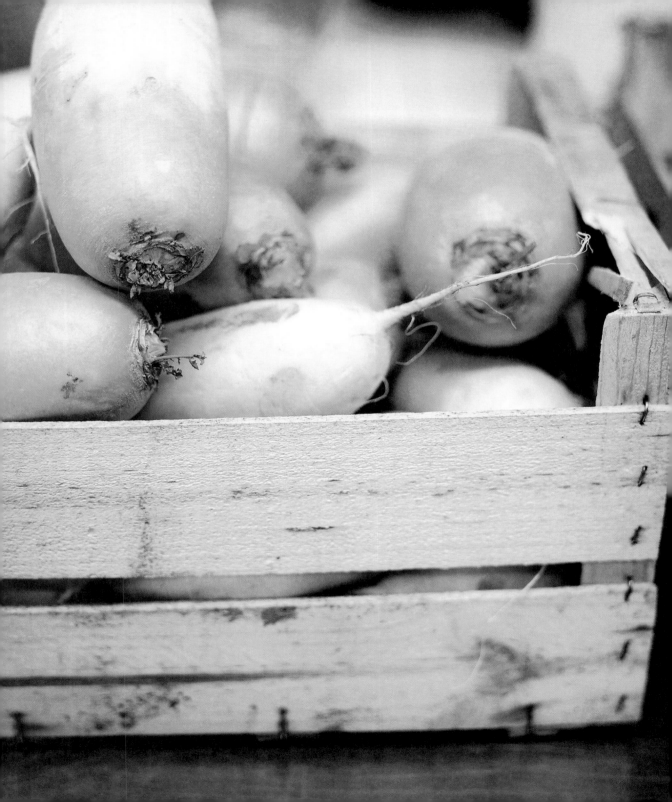

CONTENTS

THE LIM FAMILY AND ARIRANG

KOREAN KIMCHI IS neither a dish, nor a meal, nor a recipe – it is a task to be done over time. Neither is kimchi just one flavour – it is layer upon layer of flavours: hot and acidic, salty and pungent. These flavours also change, not just by virtue of the produce that was used for the particular batch, but also every time you open the lid of the kimchi jar.

The kitchen at Arirang restaurant is quiet. No hustle, no bustle, despite the crowded dining room outside. That's how the four women behind Arirang want it. Instead of the noise, it's the smells that get the attention: the simmering oxtail stock, the grated ginger, the hot steam from the rice, the pork belly being grilled.

The four family members – two sisters, one mother and an auntie – make up the heart of Arirang. The Korean restaurant on Luntmakargtan in Stockholm has been a hub for Korean food culture in Sweden for nearly 40 years. The history of Arirang began when the violin player Yoo-Jik Lim moved to Sweden from Korea in 1960 to work as a musician. At a party in Stockholm he met Im Boo Mee Ja, a Korean nurse who had just travelled to Sweden on an exchange programme. They married and had two daughters, Byung-Hi and Byung-Soon. Later their auntie Im Kee Sun came over from Korea to help look after the girls.

'It's always mum who tastes the kimchi when it's ready', Byung-Soon says. 'The whole kitchen stops for a second and everyone stands up straight and looks at mum in great anticipation. Hopefully she'll say it tastes good. Then we breathe out and get back to our work.'

Byung-Soon is stuffing halved Chinese leaf into a large plastic container in preparation for the fermentation. Not too tight but not too loose either. The more times you make kimchi, the better feel you'll get for the craft. All the steps are important, but it's not especially difficult. The challenge is to have patience – because the reward is still a couple of weeks away. ●

Kött x 20kg		
Kinakål x 6kg Gurka x 5kg Ägg x 1 låda		
Roman x 4st Isberg x 4st Mjölk x 4L M... 2kg Purjo... x 3kg	**22/8** Zapche x 17 Soja x 7 Gochujang x 12	**Bokkum sås bägare** Minitork x 2 låda Disksvamp x 10st Maskintork x 1st Handskar, L x 3st
Rättika **15kg** **på Tisdag**	Bokkum Sås 13 K n Katzu n	Sojabönor 13/9 Tofu FREDA...

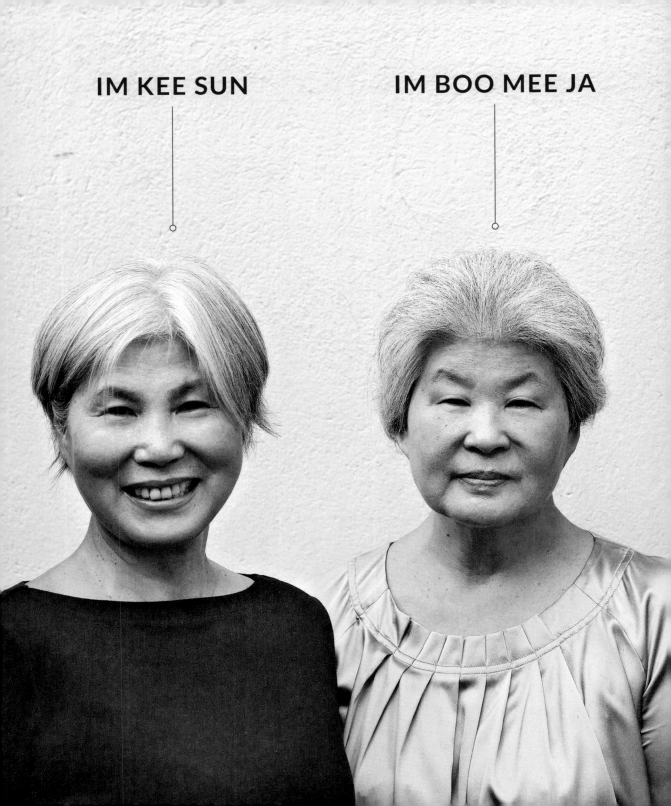

IM KEE SUN

IM BOO MEE JA

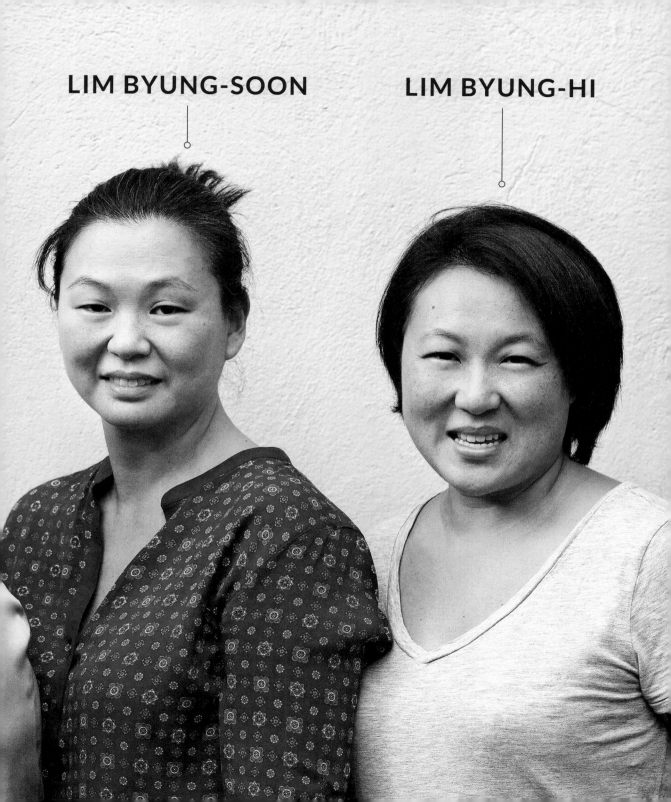

LIM BYUNG-SOON   LIM BYUNG-HI

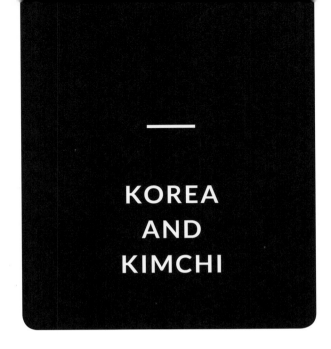

KOREA AND KIMCHI

THERE IS A Korean proverb that goes: If you have kimchi and rice – you have a meal.

The Korean table offers a lot more than just rice and kimchi, but a Korea without kimchi is simply unimaginable. Korean cuisine is a grandiose firework display for all the senses, with kimchi as the common denominator.

The secret behind Korean food lies in the contrasts of flavour and colour, of texture and temperature. From the toasted aromas of sesame oil to the sting of the chilli paste. From the freshness of the ginger to the basic notes of the garlic. The warmth from the *dolsot*, the traditional hot stone bowl, stands in even greater contrast to the Water Kimchi's cool brine. Kimchi becomes the thread that weaves all the small parts of Korean cooking together, spun from the fermented vegetables.

Many Koreans seem obsessed with kimchi; on average they eat approximately 100g of kimchi per person every day. That adds up to a lot of lacto-fermented vegetables a year, Ideally, these should be stored (free from smell) in a special 'kimchi fridge' adapted for the home. The fact that in Korea there is a public institute set up to spread the gospel of kimchi around the world (it has even been commissioned to develop a special 'space kimchi' for astronauts) seems to confirm this obsession. So, where does it come from?

Korea has four seasons, with a long, cold and stubborn winter. In the past, people had to stock up on large quantities of food in the autumn to see them through to springtime. Unlike most western cultures, despite the modernisation of homes with refrigerators, freezers and the development of chemical preservatives, Koreans have stuck with their traditional preserving methods. Still today lacto-fermentation is celebrated as the backbone of the household –

even though far from everyone in Korea still does their own fermenting.

Another explanation to the obsession with kimchi is of course its flavour. For the western palate a certain acquirement might be necessary, because the flavours of fermentation are rarely subtle. Kimchi has a bold flavour – chilli-hot with plenty of saltiness and a distinct acidity, a thoroughly umami flavour from the fish sauce and that special somewhat bittersweet experience of fermentation. Just as with truffles, kimchi is divisive, you're either not that keen – or you simply can't stop eating it.

To ferment, to let bacteria work on food, can seem a little trivial in the great world of cooking. But fermentation is actually so common that we almost stop thinking about it: bread, wine, yoghurt, chocolate, cheese, tea – in all of these very ordinary products a bacterial process is often a pre-requisite.

Fermentation is nothing strange, and the result does not have to taste like the notoriously pungent fermented herring. Kimchi is unique to Korea, but the process of lacto-fermenting vegetables pops up in many cultures around the world.

The preservation of food has historically been the crucial factor of man's survival. Fermentation is about catching the vegetable at its best and making the degradation process that follows controlled and slow, in order to create a prolonged period of use and enjoyment for us humans.

Are you ready to throw yourself into the wonderful world of fermentation? In this book you'll learn the techniques and methods to make you own kimchi, using Chinese leaf, daikon, cucumber, squash, white cabbage, carrot, oysters and ginseng, to name but a few. To embrace Korean fermentation is like opening the door to a new, healthy world full of flavour. ●

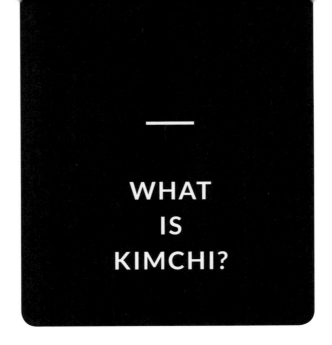

WHAT IS KIMCHI?

THE MOST COMMON kimchi recipe, *paechu*, is made using Chinese leaf, but a similar method is used for a lot of different vegetables: daikon, squash, cucumber, to name a few. It's said that there are over 200 different variations. The craft of kimchi-making in Korea is many thousand years' old, but the kimchi then looked different and didn't taste the same as today – chillies, for example, weren't introduced in Korea until the 17th century. In the same time-period, kimchi also developed to contain shellfish and fish. Traditionally, kimchi was made in late autumn, but today there are lots of varieties to eat all year round; you just use whatever produce the season offers.

Kimchi is sometimes called Asian sauerkraut, and on a bacterial level the comparison isn't completely wrong. Both kimchi and sauerkraut are fermented with help from lacto-bacteria. Unlike sauerkraut, however, the kimchi cabbage is left in a salt brine for a day before the fermentation starts. In terms of flavour, the similarities are few and far between, as the kimchi loads up on ginger, garlic, leek and Korean chilli powder. Furthermore, for the kimchi you don't only add salt, but also sugar as extra nutrition for the bacteria.

MORE THAN JUST TASTY

In Korea people pay close attention to the health benefits of food, and you often 'medicate' with help from various foods and dishes. Ginseng, algae, soya beans – everything has its own particular use. Fermented foods especially have an extra-healthy reputation due to the living bacteria culture.

Over the years, science has succeeded in identifying a number of different lacto-bacteria in kimchi, and recently a variety was isolated that's never been found anywhere else: *Lactobacillus kimchicus*. Lacto-bacteria are interesting for several reasons: they slow down the degradation process in the vegetable, force out other possibly harmful bacteria and make the raw vegetable easier to digest. The fact that kimchi also contains vitamin A, vitamin B1, vitamin B2, calcium and iron (but very few calories) makes it a good bet for those who are looking for nutritious and healthy food.

THREE STEPS TO PERFECT KIMCHI

Salting

No matter which vegetable you use, kimchi is all about creating the right environment for the bacteria to flourish and multiply. The first step in the process is to soak the vegetables in a salt brine. There are also variations where you dry-salt the vegetables, but if the kimchi is for storing over a longer period of time a salt brine is usually recommended. Sometimes it's said that the brine should be as salty as the sea, but that kind of depends on where you usually go for a swim – so do follow the measurements in the recipe and taste. Don't use salt with added iodine, as this will kill the bacteria – which in this case is counter-productive.

Note also that the amount of salt stated refers to coarse salt; if you use fine salt the end-result will be too salty.

The reason for salting the vegetables is to start breaking down the cell structure in the leaves. If you handle the leaves after the salting you'll feel that they are softer and more pliable, ready for fermenting and absorbing the flavours from the spices. Once the leaves have soaked in the salt brine they're rinsed – if not the kimchi will get too salty.

Flavouring

The second step is to make the paste that will flavour the kimchi.

At Arirang we start with leaving puréed garlic in the freezer for 24 hours. This is to make the garlic flavours a little smoother – but if you are impatient it's absolutely fine to omit this step. The garlic is mixed with grated ginger, shredded leek and daikon, and a dash of fish sauce. The fish sauce can be replaced with Korean salted shrimp or even with anchovy in brine. The idea is to give the whole thing a real kick of umami.

If you want to achieve an authentic flavour there are no excuses for not sourcing real Korean chilli powder, *gochugaru*, but of course you can make kimchi using other types of chilli powder, or without chilli altogether. The spice paste is finished off with some salt and sugar. A trick if you want the kimchi to be a little rounder in flavour is to add some rice starch diluted in water, but that's something for the more advanced course.

When you spread the paste over the vegetables you should use your hands – there are no reasons for getting any food processors out. However, plastic gloves are recommended for the novice, since chilli can be irritating on the skin. And absolutely do not touch your eyes! Make sure all surfaces of the vegetables are coated in the paste. The vegetables are then packed together fairly tightly, but without unnecessary force, into a suitable container. Use a glass jar or plastic container with a tight-fitting lid; it's important to block out any oxygen so it doesn't come in contact with the vegetables during the fermentation process. For some kimchi (e.g. Water Kimchi, see p.32 or p.46) you might need a weight to keep the vegetables submerged. For this you can use a stone (cleaned and boiled to kill off any bacteria) or a plate. Do not fill the jar all the way to the top, or it might overflow.

Fermentation

Step three is to get the fermentation started. This is done completely naturally by letting the lacto-bacteria breed at room temperature for the first 24 hours. After that you transfer your kimchi to the fridge and leave the fermentation to proceed. The lower the temperature in the fridge, the longer it will take.

After a day or two you're probably very curious to find out what's going on in the container, but do resist the temptation to open the lid. The less oxygen you let in during the fermentation, the higher the chances of a perfect result. And absolutely do not put a couple of unwashed fingers into the jar! If you are using a thinner plastic container you can often feel it bulging a little after a couple of days, once pressure has built up in there. In a glass jar you are likely to see the appearance of small bubbles. That is good news.

When the time has finally come to open the container, start by smelling. It should smell fresh, sour and aromatic. The flavour is sour as well, with a clear tang of the spices, the salt and the fish sauce. The longer the kimchi is stored, the more complex the flavours become. On the question how long kimchi will last in the fridge, mum Boo Me Ja has a great answer: 'Kimchi lasts until it's finished'. With the proviso that if it is mouldy and tastes bad, it should of course be thrown away. Within the context of fermentation, at what point something is by definition 'rotten' is a somewhat personal question, some will set the line sooner than others. Follow your own palate.

Don't forget the kimchi in the fridge just because you're not cooking anything Asian. Kimchi of course goes very well with Korean dishes, but if you make your own you'll soon realise what a versatile kitchen friend it can be. Lots of dishes can be made more exciting with kimchi: seared steak, wraps, fish and seafood dishes – the list goes on. ●

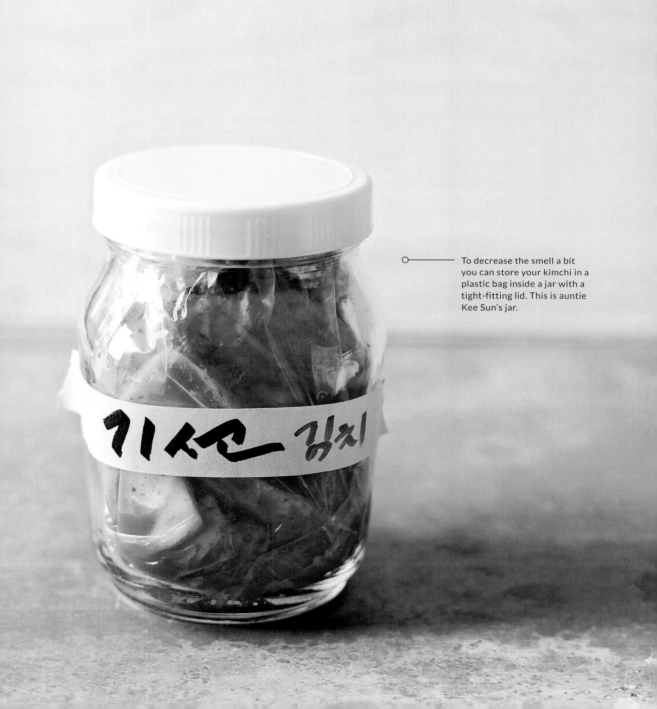

기선 김치

To decrease the smell a bit you can store your kimchi in a plastic bag inside a jar with a tight-fitting lid. This is auntie Kee Sun's jar.

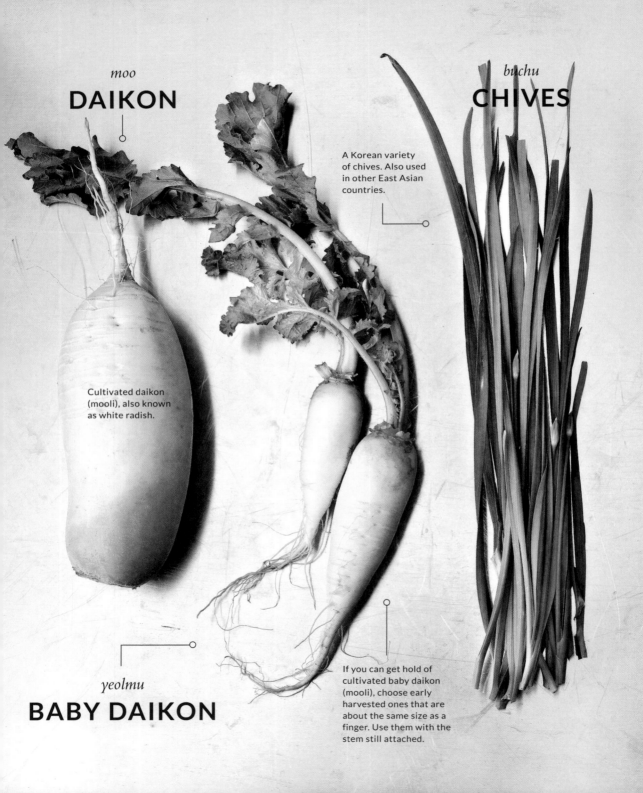

moo
DAIKON

buchu
CHIVES

A Korean variety of chives. Also used in other East Asian countries.

Cultivated daikon (mooli), also known as white radish.

yeolmu
BABY DAIKON

If you can get hold of cultivated baby daikon (mooli), choose early harvested ones that are about the same size as a finger. Use them with the stem still attached.

gochu
CHILLI

Korean green chillies are very similar to normal green chillies or very mild jalapeños. Choose a variety that is as mild as possible so that you can eat the chilli raw, together with some chilli paste for bulgogi, for example.

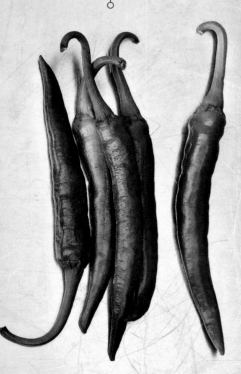

hobak
COURGETTE

Try to find small firm courgettes for Korean cooking.

oi
CUCUMBER

Korean cucumbers are firm, thin and a bit prickly.

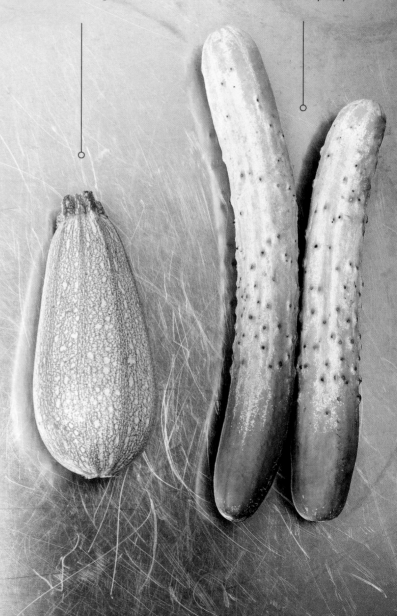

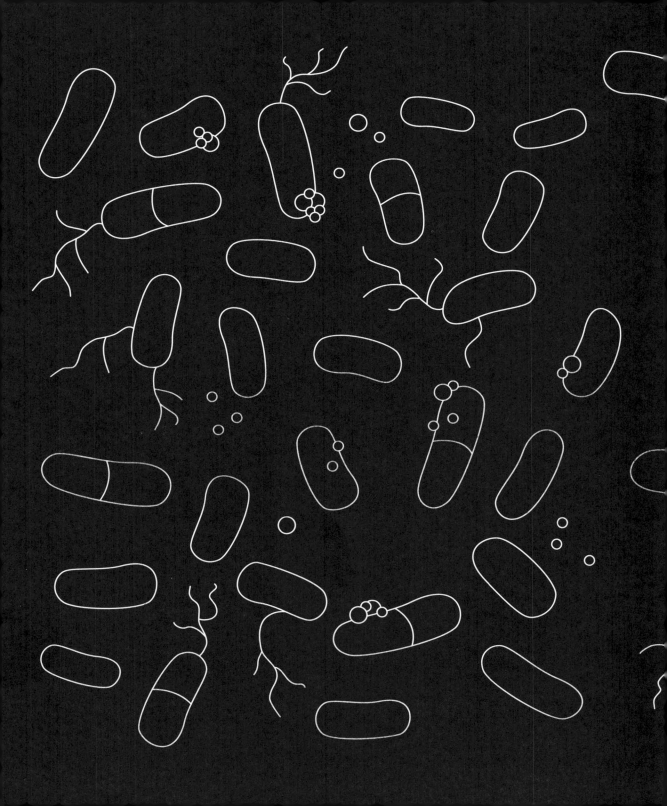

KIMCHI RECIPES

To make kimchi takes a couple of weeks, but don't let that scare you off. The actual preparation is quick and the techniques easy. The only difficult thing is to have enough patience to wait. Remember not to open the container unless necessary; during the fermentation process it will thrive best if it's left alone. The longer you leave your kimchi, the more the flavours will develop. Try as you go along and you will soon learn how 'matured' you like it. Some types of kimchi taste the best when slightly less matured, some develop complex and evocative flavours gradually. Most kimchi recipes will also work absolutely fine if you want to halve the amounts for a smaller batch.

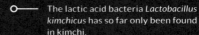
The lactic acid bacteria *Lactobacillus kimchicus* has so far only been found in kimchi.

BAECHU KIMCHI

CHINESE LEAF KIMCHI

Baechu kimchi is the most common of all kimchi varieties and the key component that is always found in Korean fridges. When you just say 'kimchi' this is the type you refer to. At Arirang batches of kimchi are prepared using twenty kilograms of Chinese leaf every other day. Korean families often have their own recipe, which of course is the best of them all. You can also halve the amounts for a smaller batch.

The art of tasting
A good kimchi contains the right amount of salt, but to get it right it's important to taste the vegetable after salting. If it's very salty the vegetable needs rinsing thoroughly. Rinse multiple times until it tastes just slightly too salty. On the contrary, if the salt level tastes just right it's probably under-salted. Adjust by either decreasing or increasing the amount of salt going into the kimchi paste.

KIMCHI RECIPES

1. Cut the Chinese leaf in half and place the halves, cut-side up, in a large bowl. Salt the Chinese leaf layer by layer (not too meticulously).
2. Pour over water so that the Chinese leaf is covered and place a plate with a weight on top, or use your kimchi stone (see p.16), so that the vegetable is completely submerged. Leave to stand for 24 hours at room temperature.
3. Drain the water and taste a bit of the Chinese leaf, preferably somewhere from the middle. Rinse the kimchi multiple times in cold water and carefully squeeze the liquid out of the leaves.
4. Mix together all the ingredients for the kimchi paste.
5. Mix the Chinese leaf and kimchi paste thoroughly. Lift and pat some paste in between the leaves.
6. Roll the Chinese leaf halves together, and place them together tightly but without too much force, with the cut-side facing up, in a jar or other container with a tight-fitting lid. Leave to stand at room temperature for 24 hours. Transfer to the fridge. The kimchi is ready after 7–10 days and will last for at least 2 months. Slice the Chinese leaf when serving.

One large jar, approx. 5 litres/8¾ pints/20¾ cups

2kg/4lb 8oz Chinese leaf
240g/8½oz/scant 1 cup sea salt

Kimchi paste
80g/2¾oz/⅔ cup *gochugaru*, Korean chilli powder
120g/4¼oz/1⅓ cups finely chopped leek
3 tbsp minced garlic
2 tbsp finely grated ginger
80g/2¾oz/heaped ¾ cup fresh daikon (mooli), shredded
1 tbsp fish sauce
1–2 tbsp salt
1 tbsp granulated sugar

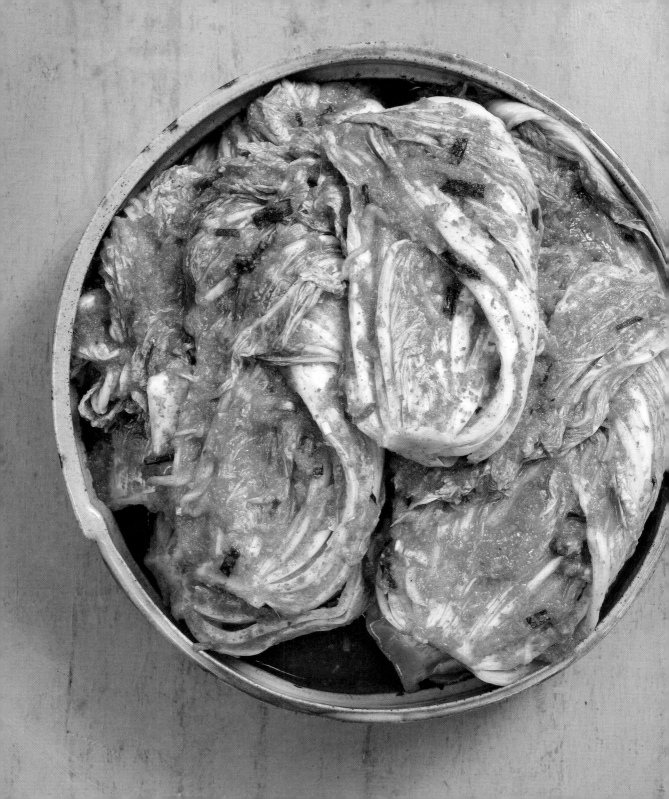

KIMCHI

Once you've made one, you'll be more or less able to make any other kimchi recipe. The process is the same for most of them, and similar for all for them.

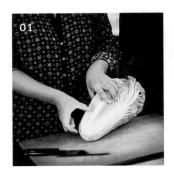

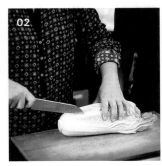

01–02. Halve the Chinese leaf at the base by making an approx. 10cm-long cut.
03. Pull the Chinese leaf apart into two halves.
04. Place the Chinese leaf in a large bowl. Salt generously, making sure a little goes in between the leaves.

05. Cover with cold water. Leave to stand for 24 hours at room temperature. Rinse the salt off in cold water. Squeeze the water out gently.
06. The Chinese leaf should be leached out but not completely mushy; it should be like a pickled gherkin, springy but soft.

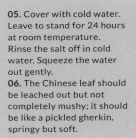

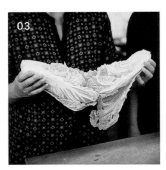

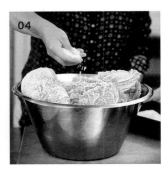

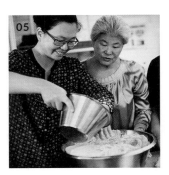

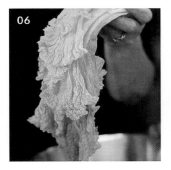

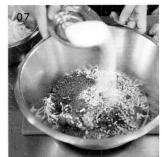

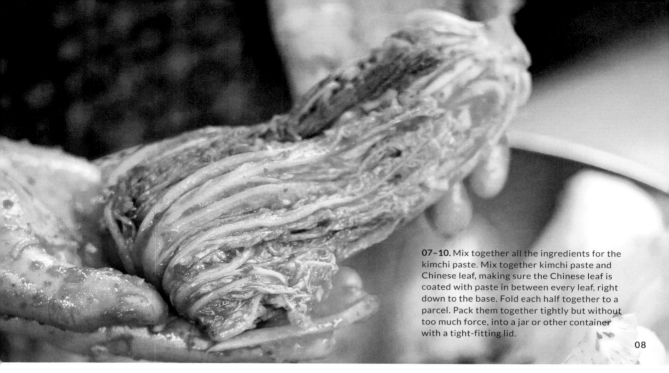

07–10. Mix together all the ingredients for the kimchi paste. Mix together kimchi paste and Chinese leaf, making sure the Chinese leaf is coated with paste in between every leaf, right down to the base. Fold each half together to a parcel. Pack them together tightly but without too much force, into a jar or other container with a tight-fitting lid.

08

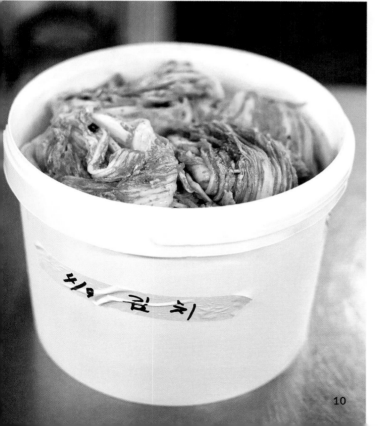

10

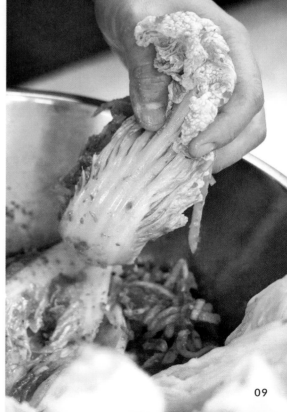

09

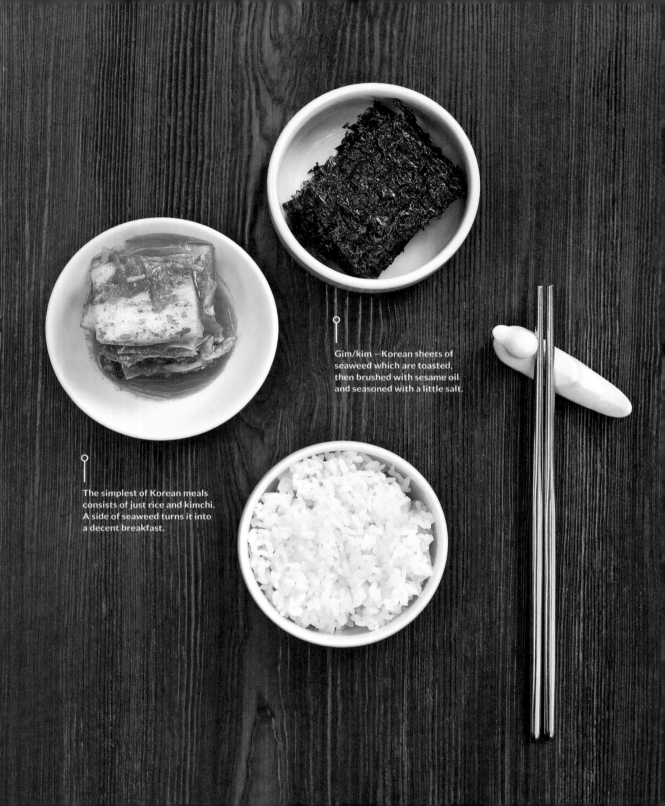

Gim/kim – Korean sheets of seaweed which are toasted, then brushed with sesame oil and seasoned with a little salt.

The simplest of Korean meals consists of just rice and kimchi. A side of seaweed turns it into a decent breakfast.

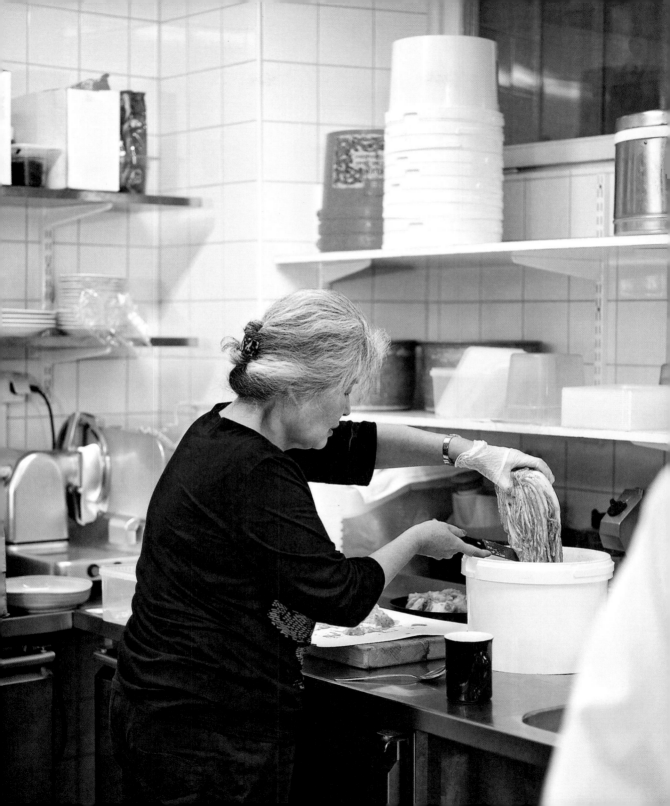

KKAKDUGI
DAIKON KIMCHI

Recognisable by the crispy crunch and acidity from the first bite. The marinated kimchi liquid that seeps through when you bite into the daikon gives you a flavour sensation that is not only chilli hot. Daikon kimchi has a completely different flavour to kimchi made from Chinese leaf. It also has a bit more sweetness than the Chinese leaf kimchi. Especially when you eat soft foods such as fish, well-marinated meat or soft delicate rice, the mouth can be in need of a contrasting texture for balance. If you can't find fresh crispy daikon it can be tricky to make this kimchi come into its own.

'The Korean way is not to blindly trust a recipe; instead they work on perfecting their 'sone mat', a Korean expression meaning 'the taste of one's hand'. Just like you get green fingers the more you work with plants, the knowledge and feeling for cooking can become set in your hands.'

1. Peel and cut the daikon into 2cm/¾in cubes.
2. Salt and cover with water. Leave to stand for at least 5–6 hours or overnight.
3. Drain the water off the daikon and check the seasoning (see p.22). Rinse repeatedly in cold water.
4. Mix together all the ingredients for the kimchi paste in a large bowl.
5. Mix together daikon and kimchi paste.
6. Place in a jar or container with a tight-fitting lid and leave at room temperature for 24 hours. Transfer to the fridge. The kimchi is ready to eat after about 1 week and will last for at least 4–6 weeks.

One large jar, approx. 5 litres/8¾ pints/20¾ cups

2kg/4lb 8oz fresh daikon (mooli)
60–120g/2¼–4½oz/scant ¼–scant ½ cup coarse
    sea salt

Kimchi paste
80g/2¾oz/scant ⅔ cup *gochugaru*, Korean chilli
    powder
120g/4¼oz/1⅓ cups chopped leek
3 tbsp minced garlic
2 tbsp finely grated ginger
2 tbsp fish sauce
1 tbsp salt
3 tbsp granulated sugar

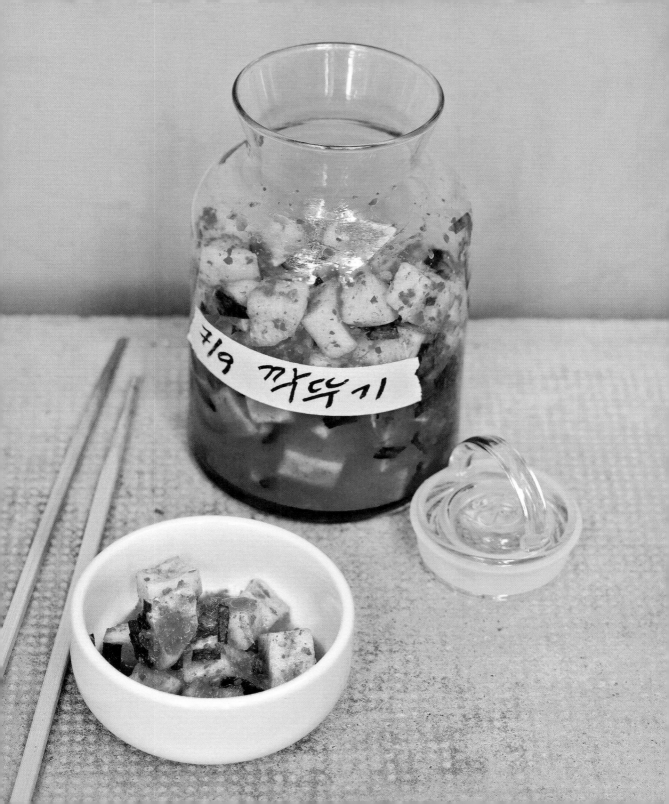

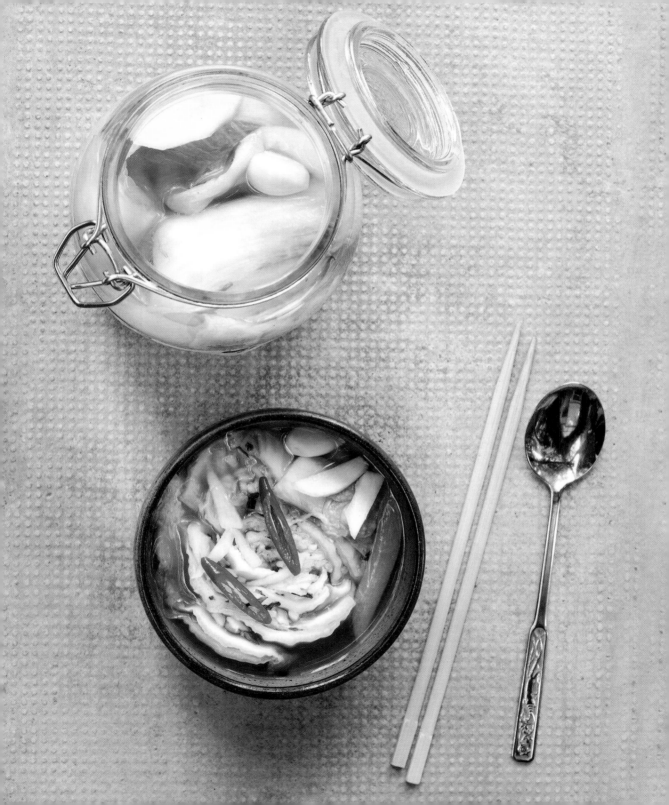

PAEK KIMCHI

WHITE KIMCHI

There are a plenty of variations of kimchi, and they don't all have to contain chilli powder or fish sauce. This kimchi is a salted and matured version with a slight acidity, but almost completely without chilli.

'As newly arrived Koreans in Sweden we did our cooking at home as we could not find it anywhere else here. When we started the restaurant we got help from our fellow countrymen — daikon for example was not available to buy, but our friends grew it for us on their allotments.'

1. Halve the Chinese leaf lengthwise. Salt and cover with water. Leave to stand for approx. 6 hours.
2. Check the seasoning (see p.22) and rinse the Chinese leaf repeatedly in cold water.
3. Make the brine for the kimchi by boiling salt and water. Leave to cool.
4. Mix together leek, garlic and ginger. Spread the spice mixture in between each leaf and press together. Place the Chinese leaf in a jar or other container with a tight-fitting lid.
5. Carefully pour the brine over the cabbage and add the whole chilli. Place a weight on top so that the cabbage is submerged in the brine. Leave in the fridge for 2 weeks. Keeps fresh for at least 4–6 weeks.
6. To serve, slice the cabbage and pour the brine into a small bowl on the side to eat with a spoon.

One large jar, approx. 5 litres/8¾ pints/20¾ cups

2kg/4lb 8oz Chinese leaf
240g/8½oz/scant 1 cup coarse sea salt
90g/3oz/1 cup finely shredded leek
1 tbsp minced garlic
120g/4¼oz.scant 1 cup finely shredded ginger
1 red chilli

Brine
3 tsp salt
500ml/17fl oz/generous 2 cups water

YEOLMU MUL KIMCHI

BABY DAIKON 'WATER' KIMCHI

In this version, early-harvested baby daikon is used. The daikon should be about the same size as a finger and is prepared with the stem still attached. The root has a deep full-bodied flavour. The small green stalk is more acidic, with a green freshness.

'When we grew up we stood beside mum in the kitchen when she made kimchi, until one day she let us do it. That is still true today. The one who is learning stands beside, until the teacher one day says "Do it yourself".'

1. Start with making rice water:
   Boil 1 tbsp cooked short-grain rice in approx. 200ml/7fl oz/scant 1 cup water until you have a white cloudy liquid. Drain off the rice grains.
2. Wash the daikon, leave the stem still attached but pick off the rougher leaves.
3. Place the daikon in a bowl, salt and leave to soak at room temperature for a few hours. Then rinse a few times in cold water.
4. Combine all ingredients for the brine. Place the daikon in a jar or container with a tight-fitting lid and pour over the brine. Store in the frige. It will be ready after about 1 week and will keep for several weeks.

2kg/4lb 8oz fresh baby daikon (mooli), preferably with leaves
240g/8½oz/scant 1 cup coarse sea salt

Kimchi brine
100ml/3½fl oz/scant ½ cup rice water (see method)
2 sliced red chillies
8 sliced spring onions
1 whole garlic bulb
30g/1oz/scant ¼ cup shredded ginger
120g/4¼oz/scant ½ cup coarse sea salt
2 litres/3½ pints/8 cups water

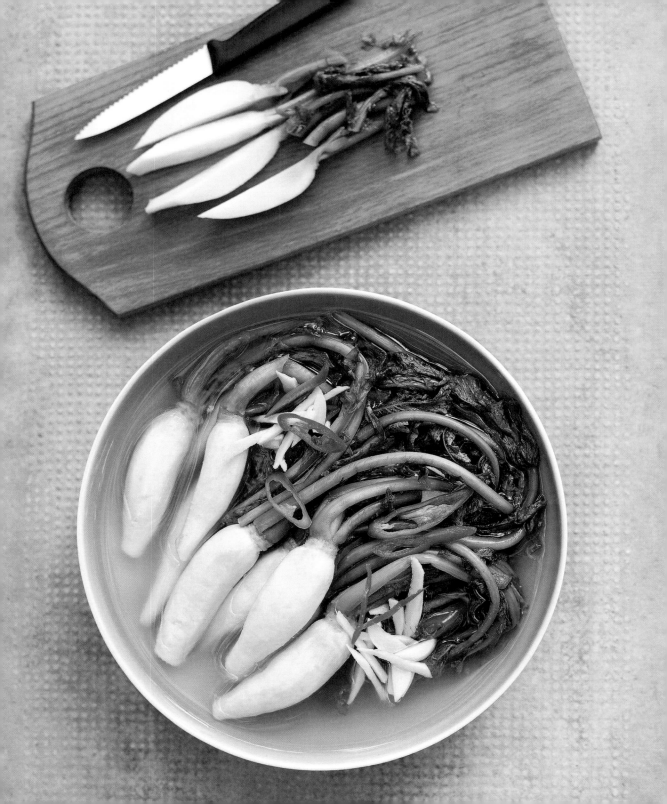

Make deep, long cuts lengthwise in the cucumber without cutting all the way through, and make sure that the kimchi paste gets into the cuts.

OI SOBAGI

WHOLE CUCUMBER KIMCHI

The crispy cucumber makes this a real fresh kimchi variety. It's tasty in all its stages, even under-fermented. It can thus be eaten straight away before it has matured. At Arirang it is especially eaten during the cucumber pickling season from July until September. Don't keep it for too long or it will go soft from over-maturing. Whole cucumber kimchi goes well with all kinds of noodles.

1. Make four cuts lengthwise in each cucumber without cutting all the way through. Salt the cucumbers liberally, making sure the salt goes into the cuts.
2. Place the cucumbers in a bowl and fill with water. Leave to stand for 1 hour at room temperature. If you are in a rush you can skip the water and just leave them to soak up the salt for 30 minutes.
3. Check the seasoning (see p.22) and rinse the salt off thoroughly.
4. Mix all the ingredients together for the kimchi paste.
5. Mix the gherkins and the kimchi paste together, trying carefully to get the paste into the cuts.
6. Place the gherkins together tightly in a jar or other container with a tight-fitting lid. Put it in the fridge. The kimchi is ready after approximately 3 days and will keep fresh for maximum of 2 weeks.

One large jar, approx. 3 litres/5¼ pints/13¼ cups

10 pickling cucumbers
150g/5½oz/½ cup coarse sea salt

Kimchi paste
50g/1¾oz/heaped ⅓ cup *gochugaru*, Korean chilli powder
80g/2¾oz/scant 12 cup finely chopped leek
1 tsp minced garlic
1 tsp finely grated ginger
40g/1½oz/heaped ⅓ cup shredded fresh daikon (mooli)
3 tbsp sea salt
2 tsp granulated sugar

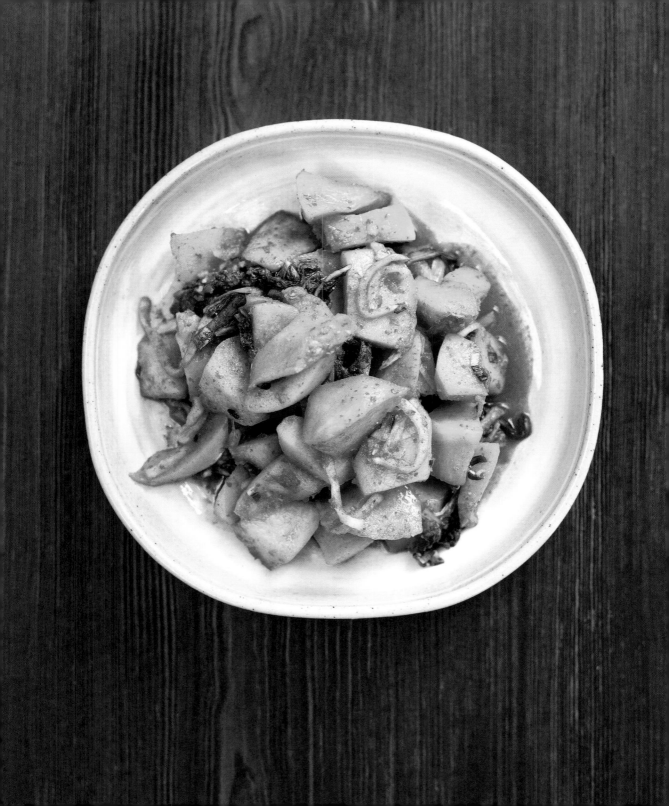

HOBAK KIMCHI

SQUASH KIMCHI

Koreans almost always refer to what a vegetable is good for. Squash in particular is said to be good for female hormones. The hard squash soaks up salt in a completely different way than, for example, cucumber, so do check the seasoning carefully. If you cannot get hold of muscat squash or butternut squash you can try a standard Halloween pumpkin.

1. Peel and cut the squash into approx. 3 x 5cm/1¼ x 1¾in pieces (5mm/¼in thick). Mix with the salt and leave to stand for minimum 10 hours at room temperature.
2. Check the seasoning (see p.22). Rinse in cold water at least two times and carefully pat the squash dry with kitchen paper.
3. Shred the Chinese leaf. Mix all the ingredients together for the kimchi paste.
4. Mix pumpkin and kimchi paste together, making sure that each piece is covered in the marinade. Place in a jar or other container with a tight-fitting lid.
5. Leave to stand for 24 hours at room temperature. Then transfer to the fridge. The kimchi is ready to eat in about 1 week and will keep fresh for at least 3 weeks.

One large jar, approx. 5 litres/8¾ pints/20¾ cups

Approx. 1.5kg/3lb 5oz muscat squash or butternut squash
480g/1lb 1oz/1⅔ cups coarse sea salt

Kimchi paste
The outer green leaves from 1 head of Chinese leaf
4 tbsp *gochugaru*, Korean chilli powder
80g/2¾oz/scant 1 cup finely chopped leek
60g/2¼oz/⅔ cup minced garlic
60g/2¼oz/heaped ⅓ cup finely grated ginger
100ml/3½fl oz/scant ½ cup fish sauce
2 tbsp salt
1 tbsp granulated sugar

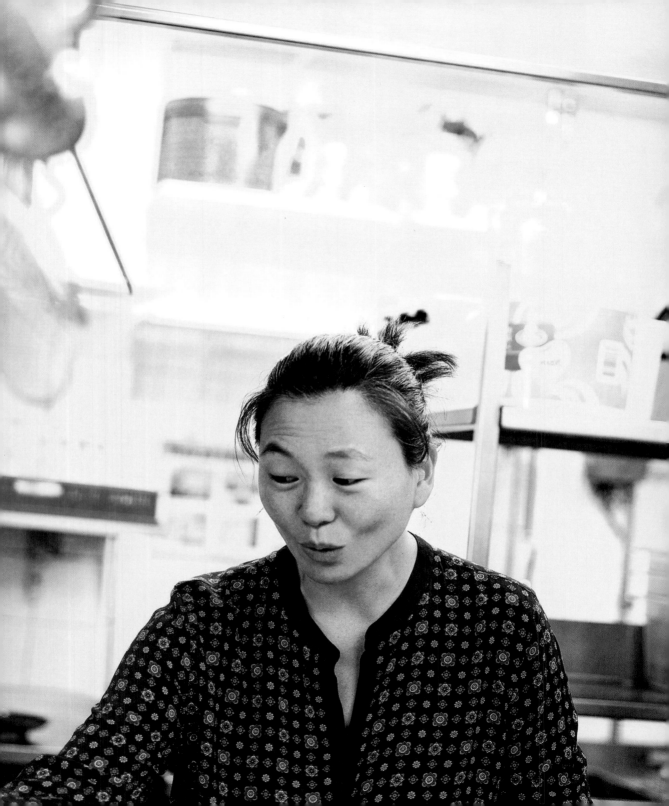

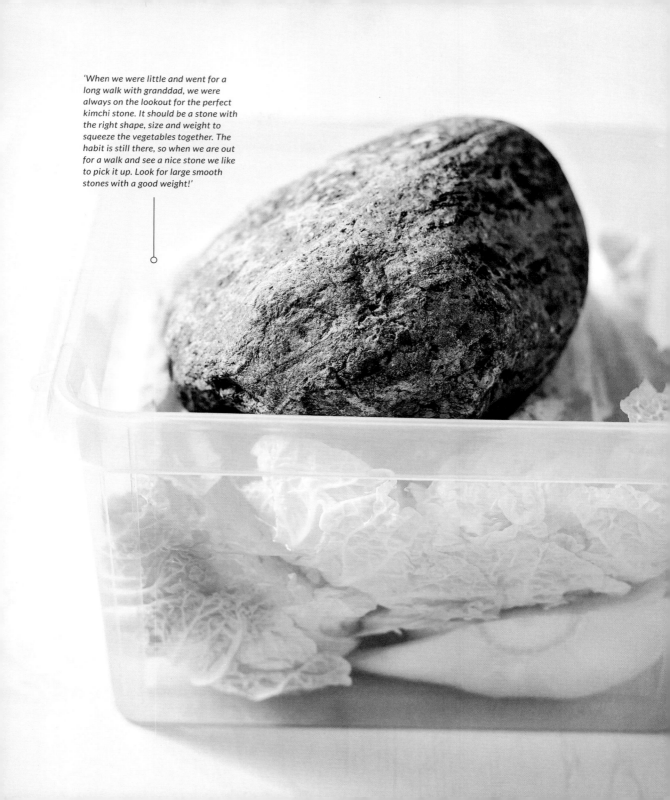

'When we were little and went for a long walk with granddad, we were always on the lookout for the perfect kimchi stone. It should be a stone with the right shape, size and weight to squeeze the vegetables together. The habit is still there, so when we are out for a walk and see a nice stone we like to pick it up. Look for large smooth stones with a good weight!'

YANG BAECHU KIMCHI

WHITE CABBAGE KIMCHI

In this recipe the kimchi is tripping into the domains of sauerkraut. Also white cabbage becomes tasty as kimchi, and, if you are to believe Korean wholefood recommendations, white cabbage can perform wonders for your facial skin. In the 1970s it was so difficult to source Chinese leaf in Sweden that Arirang replaced it with white cabbage — a lot of the guests still prefer the 'original kimchi' made from white cabbage. In this recipe you can add a little rice water (see p.32) if you want — to mellow down the cabbage aroma that can sometimes get a little strong.

1. Split the white cabbage head into four quarters and cut off the hard stem.
2. Mix salt and water and pour over the cabbage. Flip the cabbage over after 30 minutes so that the salt gets evenly distributed.
3. Take out the cabbage after another 30 minutes and rinse in cold water.
4. Mix all the ingredients together for the kimchi paste and rub it into each cabbage leaf.
5. Place the cabbage into a jar or other container with a tight-fitting lid and place a plate with a weight on top or use your kimchi stone. The kimchi is ready to eat after about 2 weeks and will keep fresh for 1–2 months. We prefer it when it has matured for some time.
6. Slice the cabbage to serve.

One large jar, approx. 5 litres/8¾ pints/20¾ cups

2–2.5kg/4lb 8oz–5lb 10oz white cabbage
120g/¼oz/scant ½ cup coarse sea salt
800ml/28fl oz/3⅓ cups water

Kimchi paste
110g/3¾oz/scant 1 cup *gochugaru*, Korean chilli powder
120g/4¼oz/1⅓ cups shredded leek
2 tbsp minced garlic
2 tbsp grated ginger
160g/5½oz/1⅔ cups shredded fresh daikon (mooli)
3 tbsp fish sauce
2 tbsp granulated sugar
1 tbsp salt

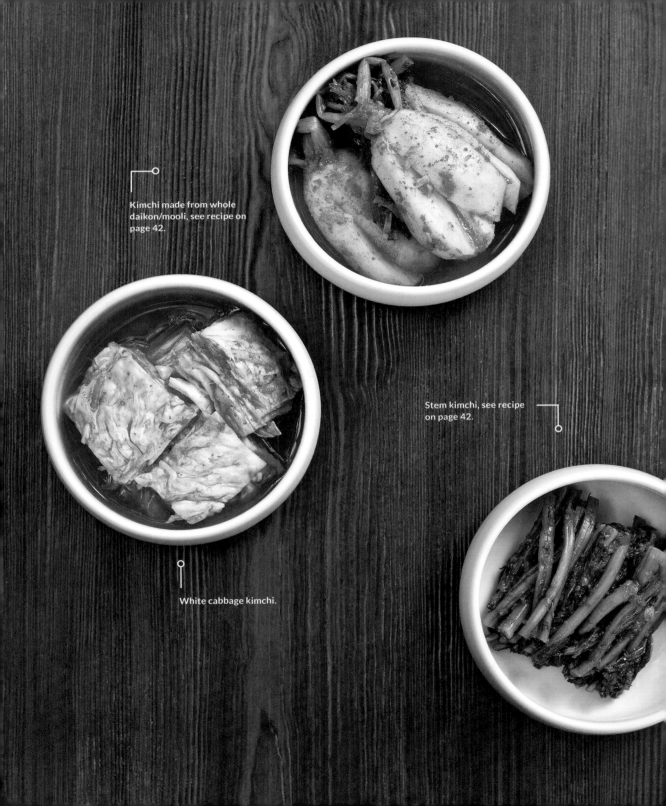

Kimchi made from whole daikon/mooli, see recipe on page 42.

Stem kimchi, see recipe on page 42.

White cabbage kimchi.

It is said that the green stems of daikon in fact contain more nutrients and fibre than the actual root. Try to always use as much as you can from the vegetable.

A summer kimchi of baby daikon. They can be hard to get hold of, so try growing your own, if possible.

One jar, approx. 2 litres/3½ pints/8 cups

1kg/2lb 4 oz fresh daikon (mooli) stems
120g/4¼oz/scant ½ cup coarse sea salt

Kimchi paste
120g/4¼oz/scant ½ cup gochugaru, Korean
    chilli powder
120g/4¼oz/1⅓ cups chopped leek
40g/1½oz/heaped ⅓ cup minced garlic
30g/1oz/scant ¼ cup grated ginger
100g/3½oz/1 cup shredded fresh
    daikon (mooli)
2 tbsp fish sauce
1 tbsp granulated sugar

1. Rinse the stems thoroughly in cold water. Place them in a bowl; add salt and splash over a bit of water (the stems should not be covered in water). Leave to stand for 2–3 hours at room temperature.
2. Check the seasoning (see p.22). Take out and rinse the stems in cold water.
3. Combine all ingredients for the kimchi paste in a large bowl. Add the stems and mix.
4. Place tightly together in a jar or other container with a tight-fitting lid. Leave the kimchi to stand at room temperature for 24 hours and then transfer to the fridge. It is ready to eat after about 10 days and will keep fresh for weeks.
5. Cut the stems into long bits before serving.

One jar, approx. 5 litres/8¾ pints/20¾ cups

3kg/4lb 8oz baby daikon (mooli)
120g/4¼oz/scant ½ cup coarse sea salt

Kimchi paste
140g/5oz/heaped 1 cup *gochugaru*, Korean
    chilli powder
40g/1½oz/scant ½ cup finely chopped leek
40g/1½oz/scant ½ cup minced garlic
50g1¾oz/⅓ cup finely grated ginger
2 tbsp fish sauce
1 tbsp salt
60g/2¼oz/scant ½ cup granulated sugar
150ml/¼ pint/scant ⅔ cup water

1. Scrub or peel the daikon. Place them in a bowl, add salt and cover with water. Leave to stand for at least 5–6 hours or overnight at room temperature.
2. Drain the water off the daikon and check the seasoning (see p.22). Rinse repeatedly in cold water.
3. Combine all the ingredients for the kimchi paste in a large bowl. Add the daikon and mix thoroughly.
4. Place the daikon in a jar with a tight-fitting lid and leave to stand at room temperature for 24 hours. Transfer to the fridge. The kimchi is ready to eat after approximately 1 week and will keep fresh for about 1 month.

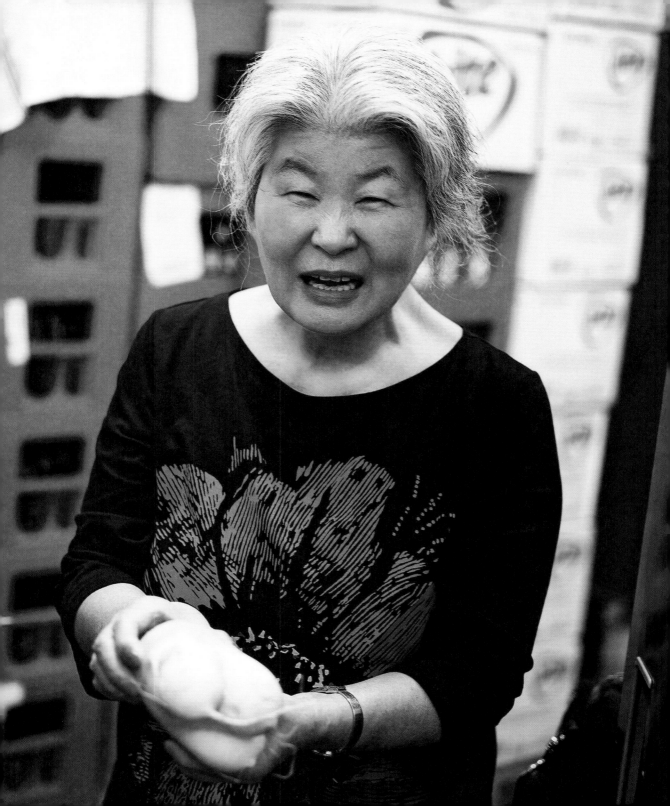

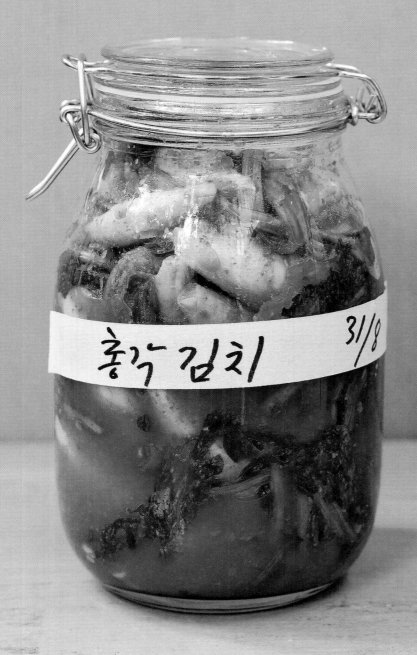

CHONGGAK KIMCHI
PONYTAIL OR BACHELOR KIMCHI

In Korean, this kimchi is called 'ponytail kimchi' since the young men of Korea a long time ago kept their hair long and tied back into a ponytail. In English it is called 'bachelor kimchi' – it is so easy to prepare that even a bachelor can manage it.

1. Salt the daikon, place in a bowl and splash over a bit or water (the daikon should not be covered in water). Leave to soak for approx. 2 hours at room temperature.
2. Check the seasoning (see p.22). Rinse the salt off in cold water.
3. Combine all the ingredients for the kimchi paste. Mix the paste and the daikon together. Grab about three daikon at a time and twist the leaves together.
4. Place the daikon in a jar or other container with a tight-fitting lid and put it in the fridge. The kimchi is ready to eat in about 2-3 weeks and will keep fresh for approximately 1 month, but tastes the best after 2 weeks.

One large jar, approx. 5 litres/8¾ pints/20¾ cups

3kg/6lb 8oz fresh daikon (mooli), preferably baby daikon with leaves still attached
120g/4¼oz/scant ½ cup coarse sea salt

Kimchi paste
140g/5oz/heaped 1 cup *gochugaru*, Korean chilli powder
40g/1½oz/scant ½ cup chopped leek
40g/1½oz/scant ½ cup minced garlic
50g/1¾oz/heaped ⅓ cup finely grated ginger
2 tbsp fish sauce
60g/2¼oz/⅓ cup granulated sugar
1 tbsp salt
100ml/3½fl oz/scant ½ cup water

DONG KIMCHI WINTER KIMCHI

Here the brine is the real delicacy. It's acidic and almost a bit bubbly. Some peeled pears are nice to include in the brine if you want to vary the flavour. Nowadays this large daikon can be sourced all year round, but in the old days, this kimchi, just like the name suggests, was made to prepare for the winter. Remember not to slice the daikon until just before serving.

Kimchi and the seasons

To make kimchi to prepare for the winter is called gimjang, and in the past it was an event where families and neighbours in the villages helped each other out – it was a big job to make enough kimchi to last for four months ahead. The older women, ajumma, often have their own tricks for making the best kimchi. Pears, apples and brine from seaweed are examples of ingredients that can be used as the icing on the cake.

1. Scrub the daikon and roll it in the salt. Place in a bowl and splash over some water (the daikon should not be covered). Leave to stand overnight at room temperature.
2. Take out the daikon and rinse it in cold water. Put it back into the bowl.
3. Bring the water and the salt for the brine to the boil. Leave to cool.
4. Peel the ginger and cut into thick slices. Peel the garlic cloves. Pick the rough leaves off the spring onion.
5. Place everything in a jar or other container with a tight-fitting lid and pour over the salt water. Put it in the fridge. The kimchi is ready to eat after about 2 weeks and will keep fresh for 4–10 weeks.

1 large jar, approx. 5 litres/8¾ pints/20¾ cups

2.5kg/5lb 10oz fresh daikon (mooli)
2.5kg/5lb 10oz/8½ cups coarse sea salt

Kimchi brine
2.5 litres/4⅓ pints/10½ cups water
100g/3½oz/heaped ⅓ cup coarse sea salt
150g/5½oz ginger
1 whole garlic bulb, peeled
10 spring onions
3 green chillies
3 red chillies

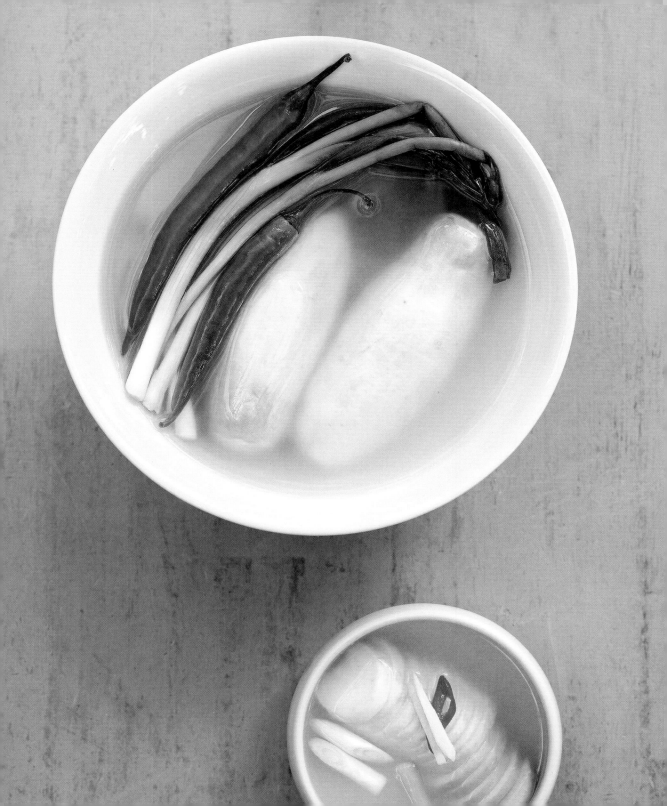

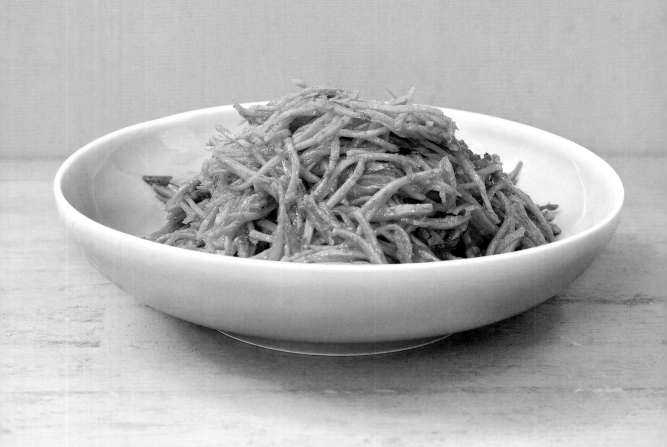

TANGGUN KIMCHI CARROT KIMCHI

Kimchi goes international. This kimchi seems to be very popular in Russia, at least it is often requested by Russian tourists who visit Arirang. The carrots can also be eaten without leaving them to ferment, but of course you'll then get a whole different flavour.

1. Peel and shred the carrots. Place them in a bowl, add salt and cover with water. Leave to stand for about 10 hours or overnight at room temperature.
2. Check the seasoning (see p.22) and rinse the carrots a few times in cold water.
3. Mix together all the ingredients for the kimchi paste. Add the carrots and mix thoroughly. Place them in a jar or other container with a tight-fitting lid. Put it in the fridge and leave to stand for 10 days. Will keep fresh for at least 1 month.

One jar, approx. 3 litres/5½ pints/13¼ cups

1kg/2lb 4oz carrots
1½ tbsp coarse sea salt

Kimchi paste
1 tbsp *gochugaru*, Korean chilli powder
20g/¾oz/scant ¼ cup shredded leek
1 tsp minced garlic
1 tsp finely grated ginger
40g/1½oz/⅓ cup shredded fresh daikon (mooli)
½ tsp fish sauce
1 tbsp salt

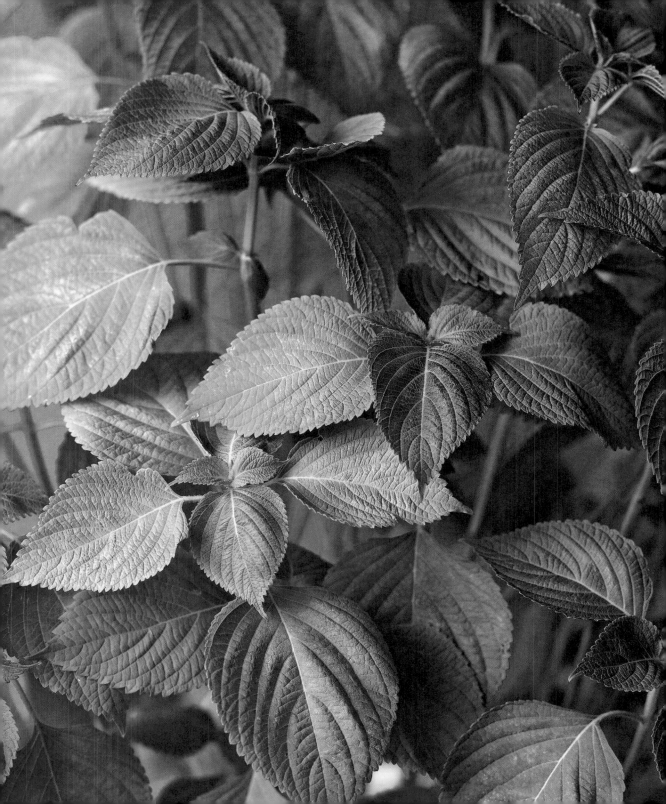

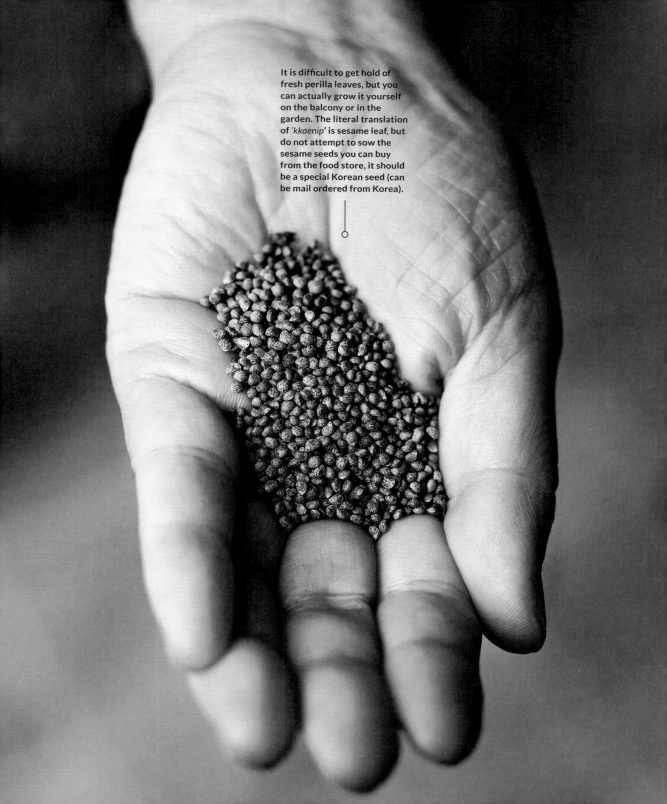

It is difficult to get hold of fresh perilla leaves, but you can actually grow it yourself on the balcony or in the garden. The literal translation of 'kkaenip' is sesame leaf, but do not attempt to sow the sesame seeds you can buy from the food store, it should be a special Korean seed (can be mail ordered from Korea).

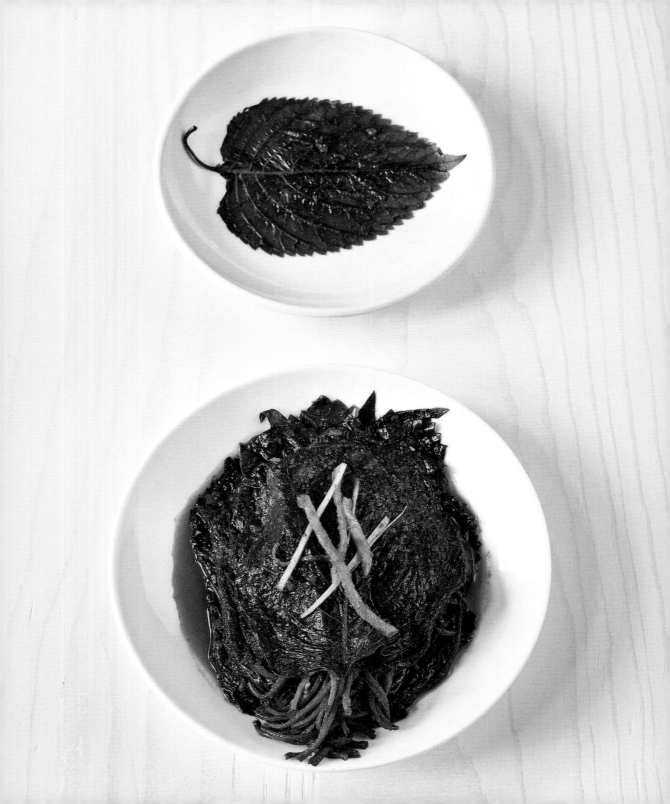

KKAENIP KIMCHI

KOREAN PERILLA LEAF KIMCHI

Korean perilla leaves have a somewhat peppery liquorice aroma and are super tasty together with grilled meat. The leaves are not to be mixed up with shiso leaves despite their resemblance. Asian food stores sell pickled perilla leaves that are tasty to eat as they are. Fresh leaves can be used for wrapping rice and other things, just like you would do with salad leaves for *ssam* (lettuce leaf wraps).

1. Mix the salt with about 200ml/7fl oz/scant 1 cup of water in a bowl and add the leaves Leave to soak for about 30 minutes. Drain and rinse the leaves in cold water.
2. Mix together all the ingredients for the kimchi paste. Spread some paste in between each leaf.
3. Place everything in a jar or other container with a tight-fitting lid. Put into the fridge. The leaves are ready to eat after 2 days and will keep fresh for 3–4 weeks.

1 side dish

100g/3½oz fresh Korean perilla leaves
90g/3oz/1 cup coarse sea salt

Kimchi paste
55g/2oz/scant 1 cup *gochugaru*, Korean chilli powder
40g/1½oz/scant ½ cup finely chopped leek
1 tbsp minced garlic
90g/3oz/1 cup shredded fresh daikon (mooli)
45g/1½oz/¼ cup granulated sugar

GUL KIMCHI   OYSTER KIMCHI

To leave a fresh oyster in the fridge for three weeks sounds like a precarious way to treat delicate shellfish, but with the added magic of kimchi that is no problem. On the contrary, oysters go incredibly well together with kimchi spices. The kind of oysters you use is not very important; any variety will make it tasty.

1. Halve the Chinese leaf lengthwise and place it with the cut side facing up in a large mixing bowl. Mix salt and water and pour over the cabbage. Leave to stand for 4 hours or overnight at room temperature.
2. Check the seasoning (see p.22). Rinse the Chinese leaf in cold water.
3. Combine the ingredients for the kimchi paste. Add Chinese leaf and oysters and mix. Try to spread the oysters evenly throughout the mixture.
4. Place everything in a jar or other container with a tight-fitting lid and put it in the fridge. The kimchi is ready to eat after about 1 week and will keep fresh for at least 3 weeks. Slice the cabbage to serve.

One large jar, approx. 5 litres/8¾ pints/20¾ cups

2kg/4lb 8oz Chinese leaf
240g/8½oz/scant 1 cup coarse sea salt
2 litres/3½ pints/8 cups water
12 oysters

Kimchi paste
115g/4oz/scant 1 cup *gochugaru*, Korean chilli powder
80g/2¾oz/½ cup chopped leek
20g/1oz/scant ¼ cup minced garlic
60g/2¼oz/scant ½ cup grated ginger
120g/4¼oz/scant 1¼ cups shredded fresh daikon (mooli)
3 tbsp fish sauce
150g/5oz/½ cup sea salt
40g/1½oz/¼ cup granulated sugar

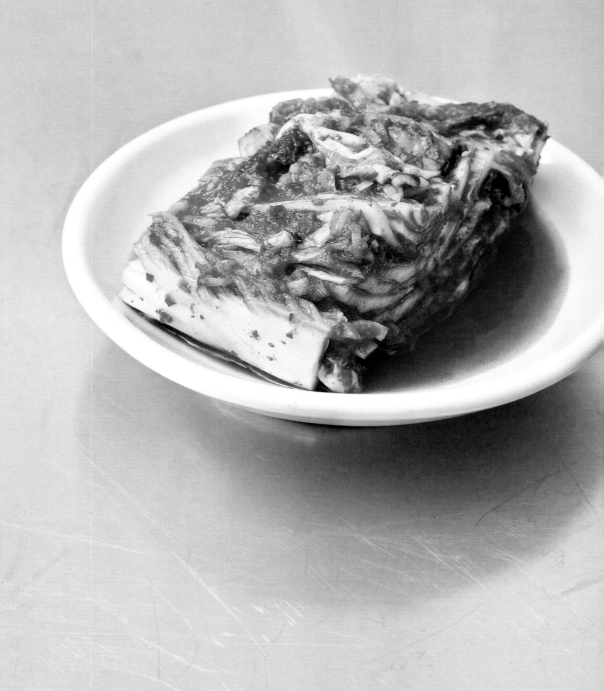

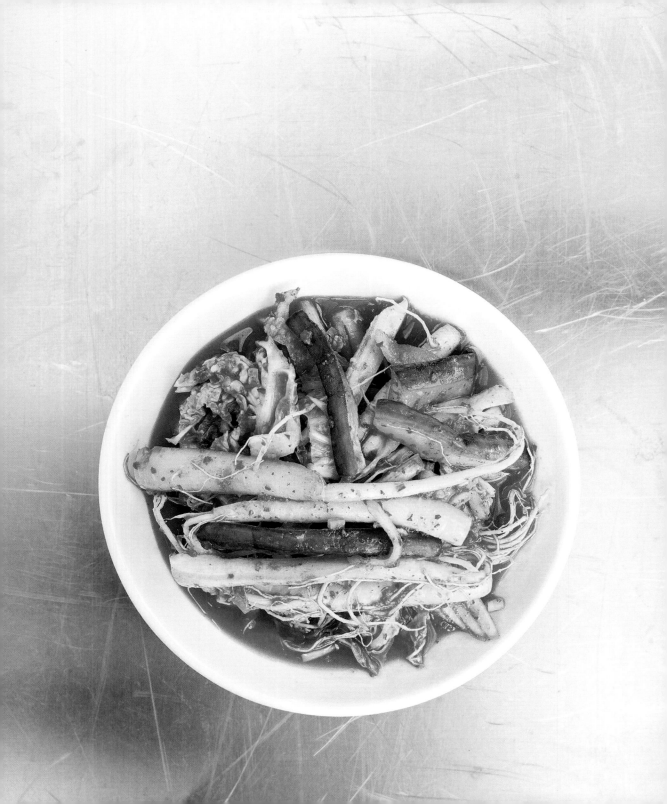

INSAM KIMCHI GINSENG KIMCHI

Many Koreans strongly believe in the salubrious powers of the ginseng root. It has been used for thousands of years and is said to help against numerous symptoms and ailments. Above all it is said to boost your energy-levels, and wild, ancient specimens are sold for large sums of money. The root almost looks like a human with legs, arms and a head. You can buy ginseng from health-food stores and some Asian food stores.

1. Cut the ginseng roots into sticks and salt carefully without damaging the bristles.
2. Cover the boiled rice with about 200ml/ 7fl oz/1¼ cups of water. Simmer until the water is cloudy and somewhat thickened. Drain, then leave the rice water to cool.
3. Slice the cucumber into sticks. Mix 100ml/3½fl oz/scant ½ cup of the rice water together with the cucumber sticks and the other ingredients for the kimchi paste.
4. Gently stir the ginseng sticks into the kimchi paste. No need to check the seasoning for this.
5. Place everything in a jar or other container with a tight-fitting lid. Put it in the fridge. The kimchi is ready to eat after approx. 10 days and will keep fresh for at least 2 months.

One jar, approx. 2 litres/3½ pints/8 cups

Approx. 20 (300g/10½oz) thin fresh ginseng roots
120g/4¼oz/scant ½ cup coarse sea salt

Kimchi paste
30g/1oz/¼ cup cooked short-grain rice
½ cucumber
110g/3¾oz/scant 1 cup *gochugaru*, Korean chilli powder
40g/1½oz/½ cup finely chopped leek
2 tbsp minced garlic
1 tbsp finely grated ginger
40g/1½oz/heaped ⅓ cup shredded fresh daikon (mooli)
30g/1oz/scant ½ cup Chinese leaf, the white part
¼ Savoy cabbage
100ml/3½fl oz/scant ½ cup fish sauce
2 tbsp salt
2 tbsp granulated sugar

When making quick kimchi, for a swift parboil you can pour boiling water over the cabbage before rinsing and mixing it with the other ingredients.

참기

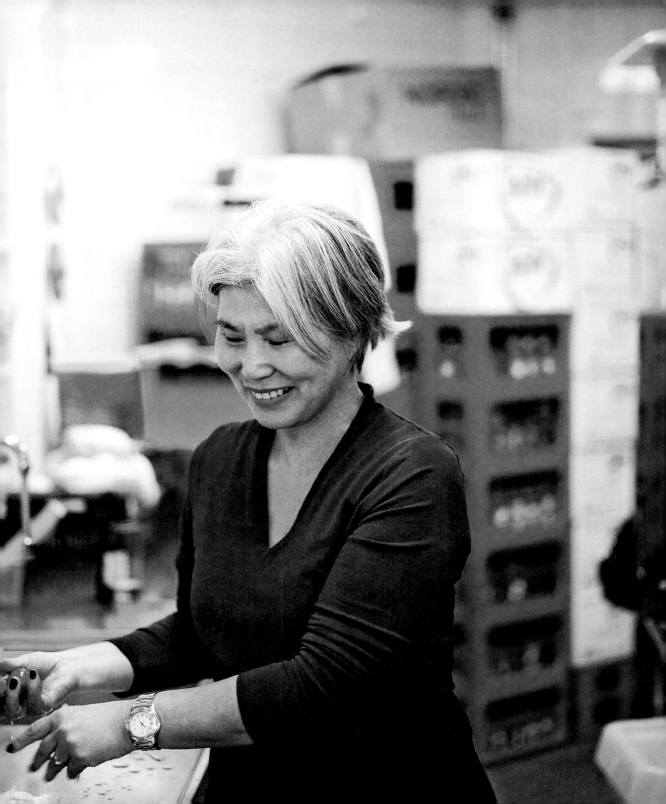

GEOTJEORI KIMCHI QUICK KIMCHI

Fancy a bit of kimchi but haven't got the patience to wait until the fermentation of the proper batch is ready? Make this recipe which you can eat straight away and where the vinegar contributes the acidity instead of the fermentation process. Speaking of quick kimchi, here is a tip: when you have salted the vegetables for a large batch of Chinese leaf kimchi and then rinsed it in water, you often end up with a few bits of Chinese leaf scraps. Squeeze the water out of it and mix with some kimchi paste, sesame oil, vinegar and sugar, add some shredded cucumber and you have quickly made a fresh salad.

'When we were little there was no Chinese leaf to get hold of in Sweden. Occasionally we would get a large batch delivered by a lorry from the continent. There were times when we had to salt the Chinese leaf in the bathtub — the only bowl that was big enough.'

KIMCHI RECIPES

1. Halve the Chinese leaf. Place it in a large mixing bowl and salt. For the best result, place a kimchi stone or other weight on the Chinese leaf so that it is pressed together. Wait for a few hours.
2. Rinse the Chinese leaf in cold water and chop it into pieces. Slice the cucumber thinly. Roughly chop the spring onions.
3. Mix together all the ingredients for the kimchi paste. Add Chinese leaf, cucumber and spring onions. Stir and sprinkle some sesame seeds on top.

1 large bowlful

2kg/4lb 8oz Chinese leaf
240g/8½oz/scant 1 cup coarse sea salt
½ cucumber
3 spring onions

Kimchi paste
5 tbsp *gochugaru*, Korean chilli powder
3 tbsp minced garlic
2 tbsp grated ginger
about 150g/5oz/1¾ cups shredded fresh daikon (mooli)
1 tbsp fish sauce
100ml/3½fl oz/scant ½ cup sesame oil
5 tbsp distilled vinegar, 12%
5 tbsp granulated sugar

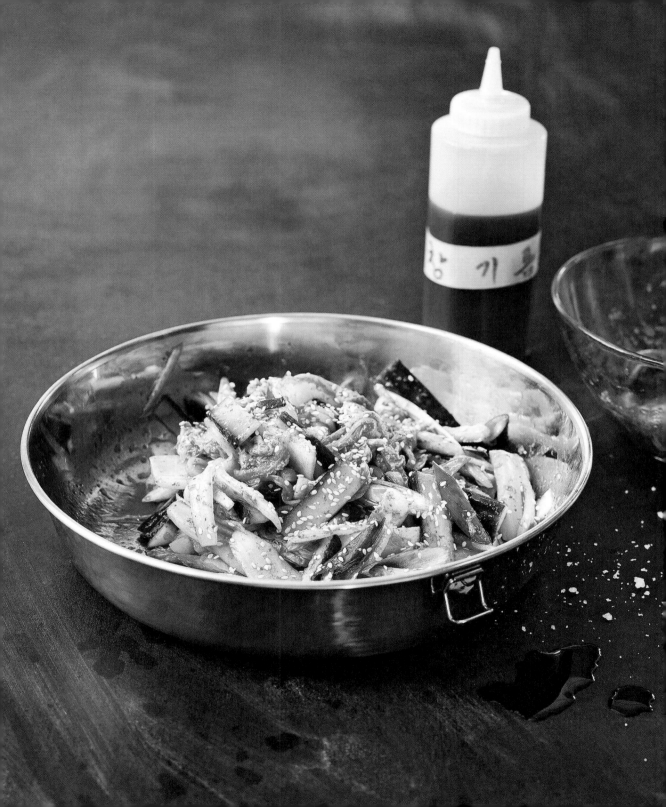

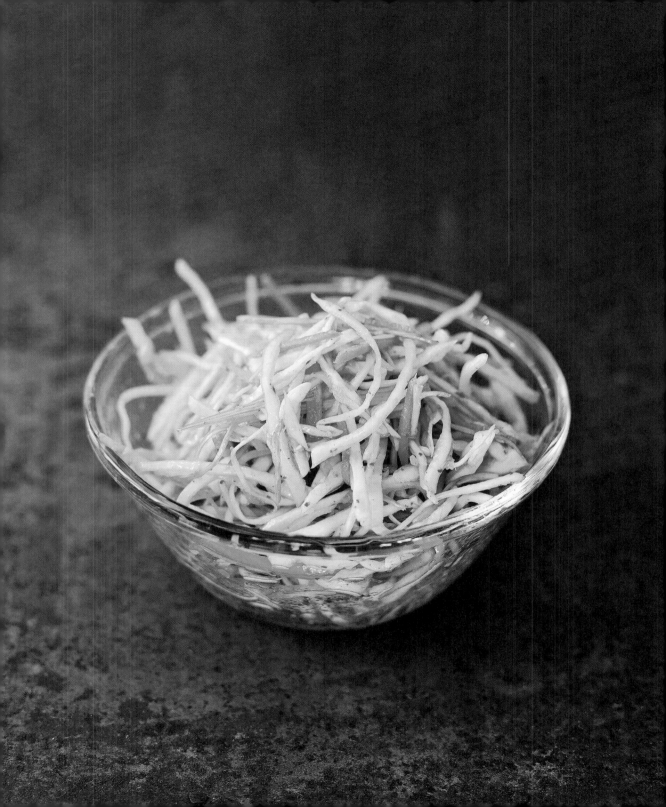

COLESLAW KIMCHI

A delicious take on classic coleslaw but without the mayonnaise and with more of a kick to it. Goes perfectly with a piece of grilled fish or meat, on your sandwich or as a side dish. Together with a few green leaves and some veg the coleslaw is quickly transformed into a filling salad.

1. Shred the white cabbage and mix together with the leek and carrot in a bowl.
2. Add the other ingredients and mix. Can be eaten straight away and will keep fresh in the fridge for 1 week.

Serves 4

Approx. 600g/1lb 5 oz white cabbage
90g/3oz/1 cup finely shredded leek
45g/1½oz/⅓ cup finely shredded carrot
2 tbsp *gochugaru*, Korean chilli powder
1 tsp minced garlic
1 tsp finely grated ginger
1 tbsp distilled vinegar, 12%
2 tbsp sesame oil
1–2 tsp salt
½–1 tbsp granulated sugar

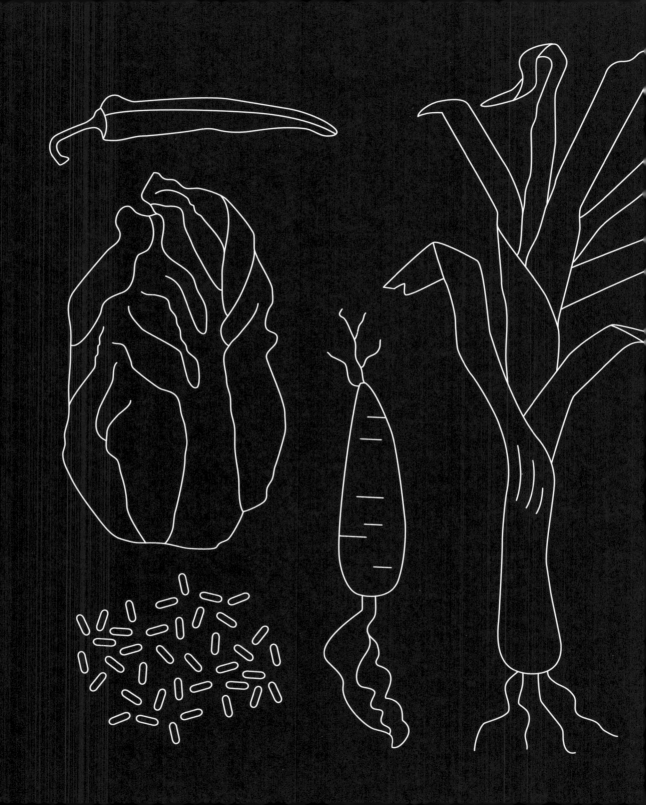

KIMCHI IN FOOD

Kimchi is a lot more than just a side dish for the table. In soups, noodle dishes, Korean pancakes or dumplings, kimchi becomes both a substantial ingredient and a versatile spice. Even if your kimchi over time has become a bit too acidic to be eaten as a side dish it can be perfect for cooking. Remember that, if required, you can rinse off the leaves and slice them up to be used in stews or soups.

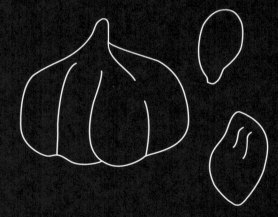

A lot of the kimchi's acidity sits in the brine. If you cook kimchi the acidity disappears and is instead replaced with the naturally occurring sugars within the vegetable itself.

KIMCHI JJIGAE

KIMCHI SOUP

Kimchi soup is a true comfort food for Koreans. A food cuddle that cures all types of homesickness. Want to make the kimchi soup vegetarian? Swap the meat for more tofu and use a vegetarian stock.

1. Cut the pork collar into thin strips and the tofu into cubes or thick domino tiles.
2. Brown off the meat in some oil in a pan over medium heat. Add the kimchi and fry for about another 5 minutes.
3. Add the water and bring to the boil. Turn down the heat and leave the soup to simmer without a lid for about 10 minutes.
4. Add leek and tofu, leave to simmer for a minute or so more. Finish off by adding sesame oil to taste. Serve with a bowl of rice on the side.

Serves 4

200g/7oz pork collar
250g/9oz firm tofu
300–400g/10½–14oz/2½–3⅓cups sliced
    Chinese leaf kimchi, see p.22
800ml/28fl oz/3⅓ cups water
45g/1½oz/½ cup chopped leek or spring onions
Approx. 1 tbsp sesame oil
cooking oil for frying

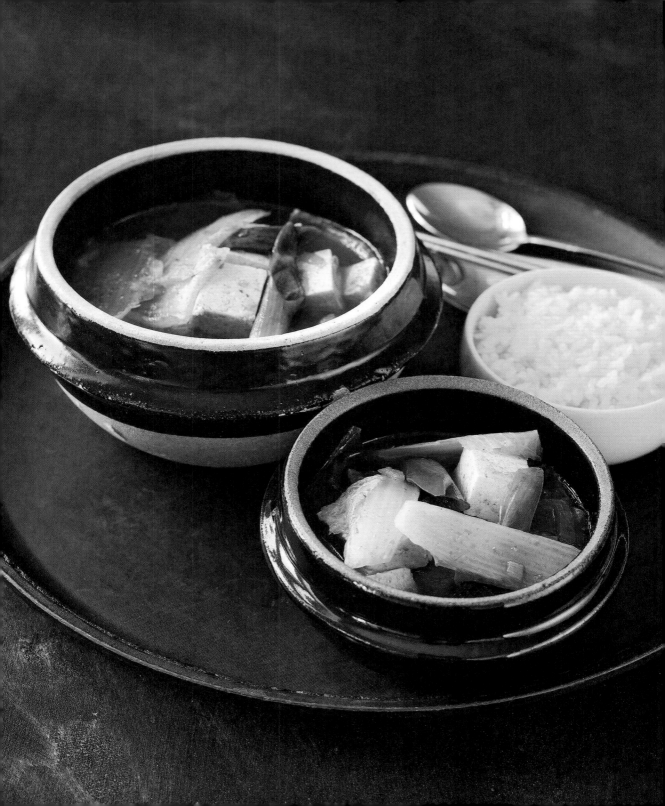

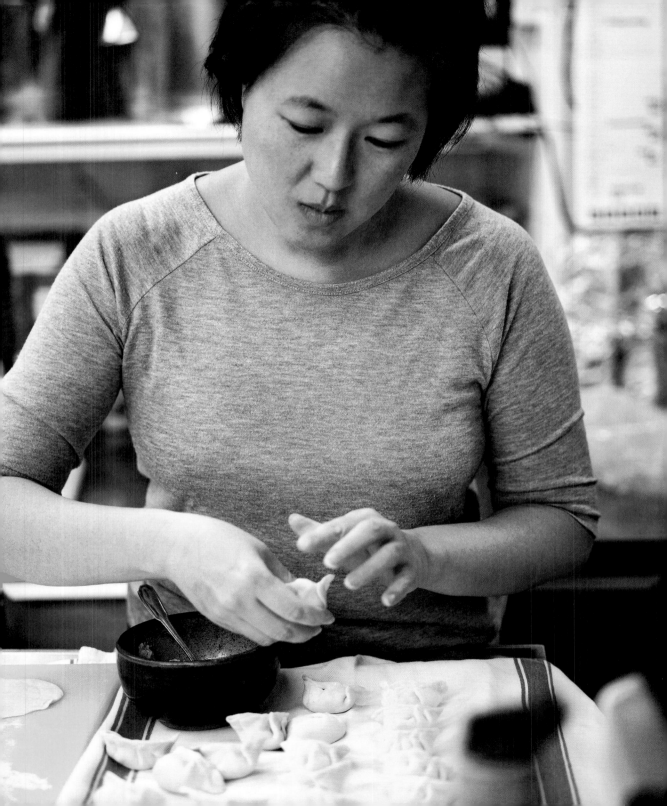

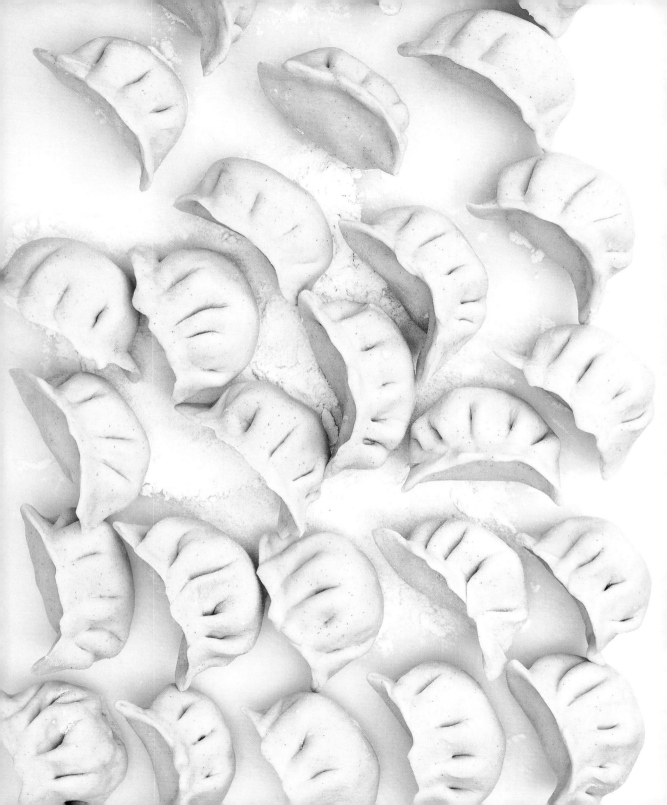

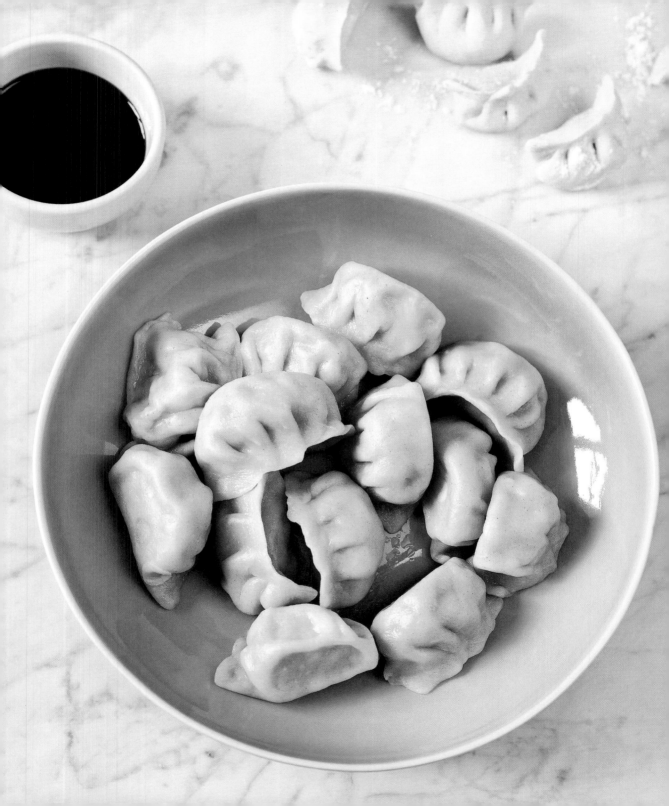

KIMCHI MANDU

KIMCHI DUMPLINGS

This is Arirang's version of dumplings. Remember to squeeze out the liquid from the kimchi so that the filling doesn't get too watery. This recipe is good for making a large batch to put in the freezer. Leftover *mandu* are also very tasty fried until crispy in a little oil.

1. Mix together all the ingredients for the mince.
2. Combine flour and water to a firm dough. Roll out the dough to 5–8 thin strips and cut every strip into 2cm/¾in squares. Form each square into a ball and roll out onto a lightly floured work surface. Be careful not to use too much flour or it will be difficult to get the edges to stick together. Roll every ball out to a thin disc, approx. 7–8cm/2¾–3¼in.
3. Place about 1 tbsp of filling in the middle of each disc. Stick together the edges by forming the dough into small crimps that you press down gently. Fold every disc into a half-moon shape.
4. Mix together the ingredients for the dipping sauce.
5. Place the *mandu* in boiling water and simmer for 6–7 minutes until cooked through. If you have a large pan you can boil all in one go, if not do a few at a time. Take out the *mandu* and eat straight away, together with the dipping sauce.

Serves 3–4

200g/7oz coarse ground pork
50g/1¼oz lard or ground pork with as high fat content as you can find
20g/¾oz/scant ¼ cup finely chopped leek
1½ tbsp grated ginger
40g/1½oz/1 cup finely chopped brown onion
30g/1oz/¼ cup parboiled and finely chopped white cabbage
50g/1¾oz/½ cup Chinese leaf kimchi, with the liquid squeezed out, see p.22
1 tbsp sesame oil
salt and black pepper

Dough
350g/11oz/scant 3 cups plain flour
200–240ml/7–8fl oz/scant–1 cup water

Dipping sauce
3 tbsp Korean or Japanese soy sauce
½ tbsp sesame oil
1 dash distilled vinegar, 12%

KIMCHI MANDU

STEP-BY-STEP

'Some of our earliest memories of dad are when he took out the pasta machine to make mandu. *We helped pulling out metre-long pasta sheets which we then cut out to round pasta discs. What really made it fun was that we all converged and cooked food together. Nowadays we use a rolling pin, but that doesn't make making mandu any less fun.'*

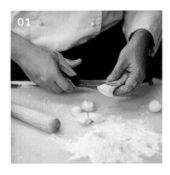

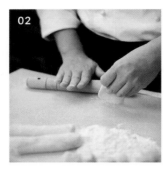

01. Make the dough and roll it out to thin strips. Cut each strip into squares.
02. Form each square into a ball and roll out on a lightly floured surface.

03-07. Place about 1 tbsp of filling on each dough disc. Fold into a half-moon shape by making small crimps in the dough along the edge which you gently press down.

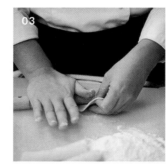

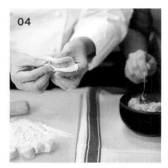

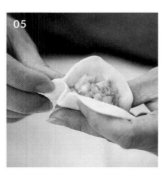

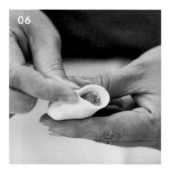

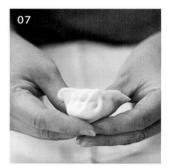

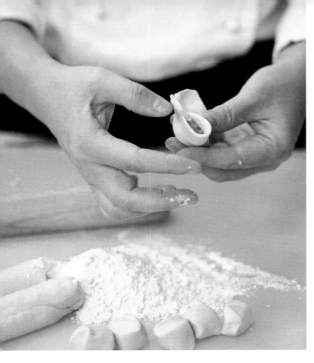
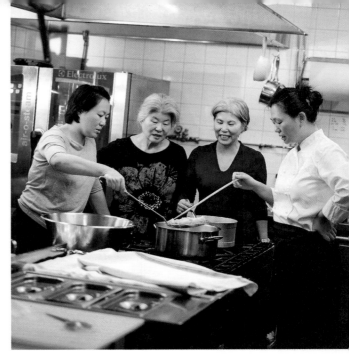
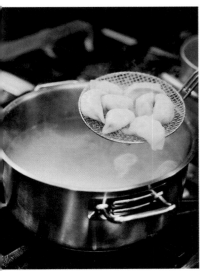
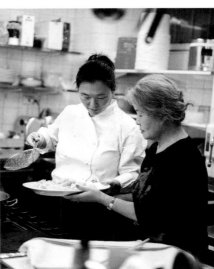
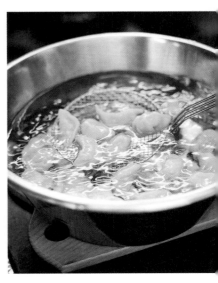
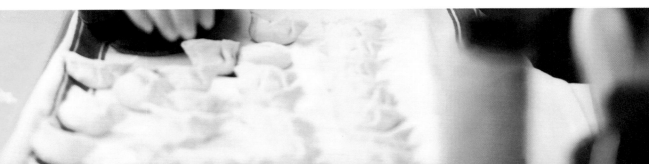

CONDIMENTS

KIMCHI BUTTER

Use in the same way as herb butter and add
a bit on top of your fried pork chop or fry the
meat directly in the butter.

1. Mix together butter, kimchi and chilli paste.
   Place the kimchi butter on a sheet of clingfilm
   and shape into a sausage. Leave in the fridge for
   a little while.
2. Take it out and slice into 1cm/¾in thick slices.

Makes 100g/3½oz

100g/3½oz unsalted butter
2 tbsp finely chopped Chinese leaf kimchi,
    with the liquid squeezed out, see p.22
1 tbsp *gochujang*, Korean chilli paste

KIMCHI DRESSING WITH EGG

The egg makes the dressing a little thicker and
more robust in flavour and will bind together
salads with large broad leaves more easily.

1. Mix together all the ingredients and whisk into
   a dressing. Season with salt and sugar. Garnish
   with chilli powder (optional).

Makes 300ml/½ pint/1¼ cups

4 tbsp kimchi brine
200ml/7fl oz/scant 1 cup sesame oil
1 egg yolk
1 tbsp white wine vinegar
1 tsp granulated sugar
½ tsp salt

KIMCHI DRESSING

An outstanding way to make use of the
kimchi brine.

1. Mix together all the ingredients and whisk into
   a dressing. Taste to check whether you will
   need more sugar and salt.

Makes 300ml/½ pint/1¼ cups

5 tbsp kimchi brine
200ml/7fl oz/scant 1 cup sesame oil
1 tbsp white wine vinegar
1 tsp granulated sugar
1 pinch salt

KIMCHI MAYONNAISE

Now we are going to make it easy for
ourselves and let everyone use whichever
mayonnaise they want – whether it is bought
or homemade.

1. Mix together mayonnaise, kimchi paste and
   kimchi. Add sesame oil during whisking.

Makes 300ml/½ pint/1¼ cups

200ml/7fl oz/scant 1 cup mayonnaise
4 tbsp kimchi brine
2 tbsp finely chopped Chinese leaf kimchi with
    the liquid squeezed out, see p.22
2–3 tbsp sesame oil

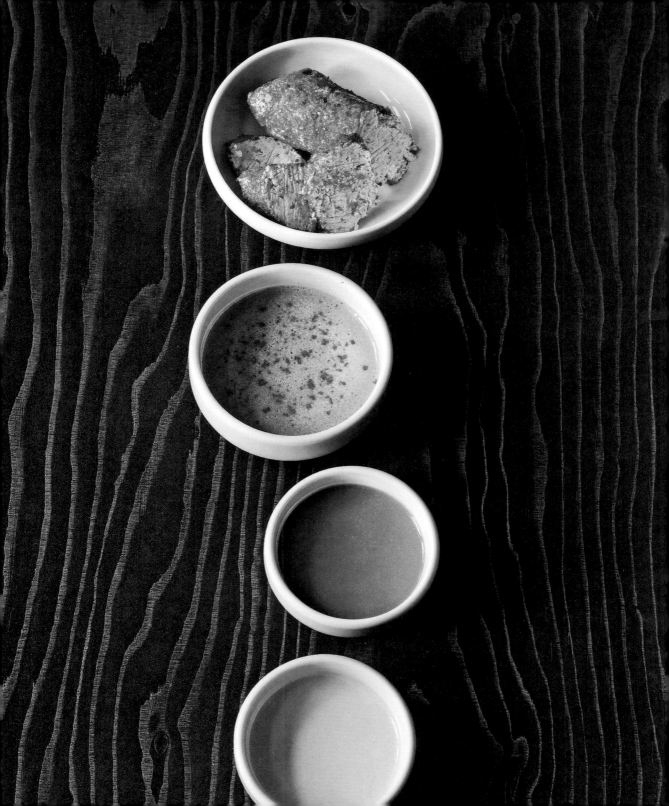

KIMCHI KIMBAP

KIMCHI ROLLS

Deceptively similar to Japanese *maki* rolls, but the Korean *kimbap* is something completely unique. In this recipe, rice and seaweed encase bulgogi meat, but the filling can also be made up of fish or vegetables. Tip: try dripping a few drops of distilled vinegar and sprinkling some granules of sugar over the newly boiled rice.

1. Whisk together the eggs and fry them as you would an omelette, in a frying pan over medium heat. Leave to cool slightly and then cut into long strips. Shred the bulgogi.
2. Place a sheet of seaweed onto a rolling mat. Spread a layer of rice over half of the sheet.
3. Place meat, kimchi and omelette in a thin line on top of the rice.
4. Roll together into a firm roll with help from the mat. 'Glue' the edge of the sheet together using a few rice grains or some water. Place with the seam facing down and slice into bite-sized rounds.

4 rolls

2 eggs
4 seaweed sheets for sushi
200g/7oz/heaped 1½ cups cooked short-grain rice
150g/5½oz bulgogi, see p.106
110g/3¾oz/1 cup shredded kimchi

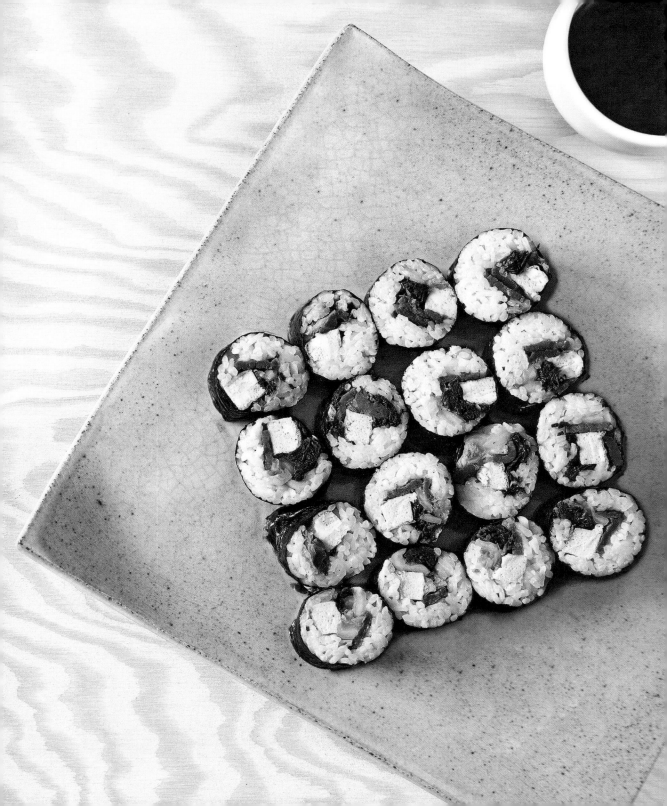

KIMCHI KIMBAP

In Korea *kimbap* is the ultimate picnic food. Start by preparing and slicing all the ingredients finely.

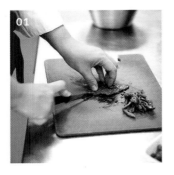

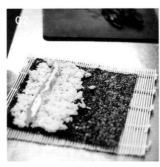

01. Slice all the vegetables and the meat into long thin strips.
02. Place a seaweed sheet onto a rolling mat. Spread out an approx. 1cm/½in-thick layer of cooked rice on one half of the sheet. Place the shredded vegetables and the meat in a thin line on top of the rice.

KIMCHI IN FOOD

03–05. Only use a little bit of each ingredient, or the roll will become too thick. You should be able to eat them in one mouthful, so try to make them bite-sized.
06–08. Form into a firm roll with help from the rolling mat.

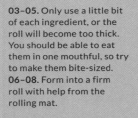

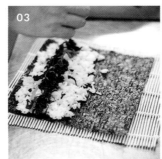

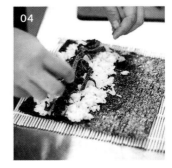

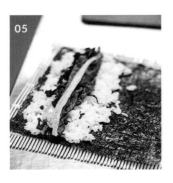

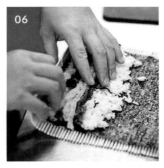

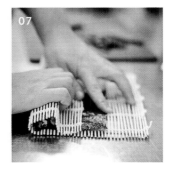

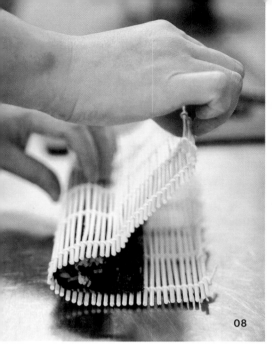

08

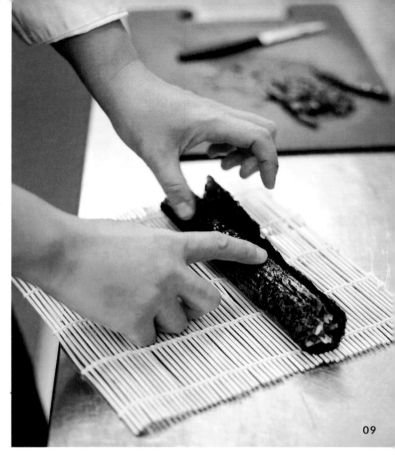

09

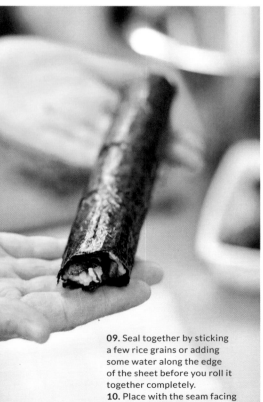

09. Seal together by sticking a few rice grains or adding some water along the edge of the sheet before you roll it together completely.
10. Place with the seam facing down and slice into bite-sized rounds.

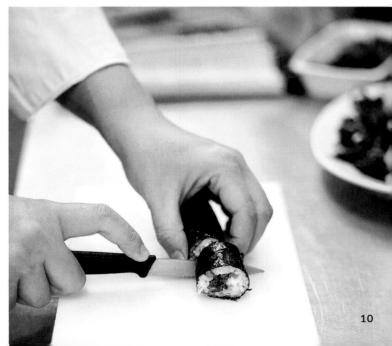

10

KIMCHI BAP

KIMCHI RICE

Bap means rice in Korean, and more complicated than that this dish doesn't have to be. To leave kimchi to cook into the rice will make it both savoury, filling and tasty. The Spanish have *paella*, the Indians have *biryani* and the Koreans have *kimchi bap*.

'Us sisters have grown up with the restaurant. After school we came straight here, helped peeling some onions, putting away some dishes and then sat down with our homework. Fermenting vegetables is something that our family has done for our whole lives.'

1. Rinse the rice thoroughly in cold water.
2. Fry kimchi, sugar, sesame oil and leek in a frying pan over a medium heat. Leave to cool slightly.
3. Place the rice in a pan or rice cooker and put the kimchi mixture on top of the rice. Carefully pour over the water. Cover with a lid and bring to the boil. Turn down the heat to half after about 6 minutes. Turn down again to the lowest setting after 6–10 minutes. Turn the heat off and leave to rest for a few minutes with the lid still on before serving. Mix together the ingredients for the soy sauce and serve together with the rice.

Serves 4

480g/1lb 1oz/2½ cups short-grain rice
200g/7oz/scant 2 cups shredded Chinese leaf
    kimchi, see p.22
2 tbsp granulated sugar
2 tbsp sesame oil
4 tbsp finely chopped leek
600ml/1 pint/2½ cups water
cooking oil for frying

Soy sauce
2 tbsp Korean or Japanese soy sauce
1 tsp sesame oil
1 tbsp sliced spring onion

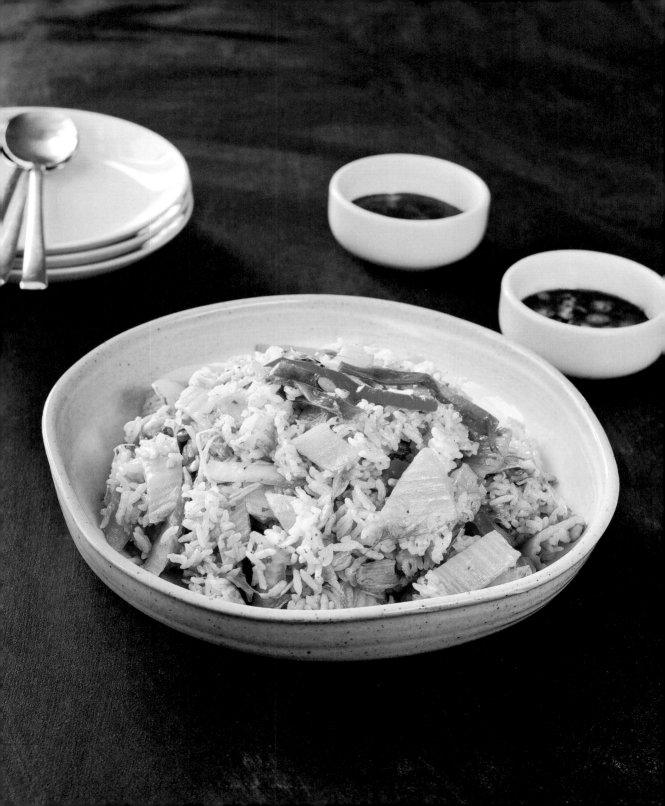

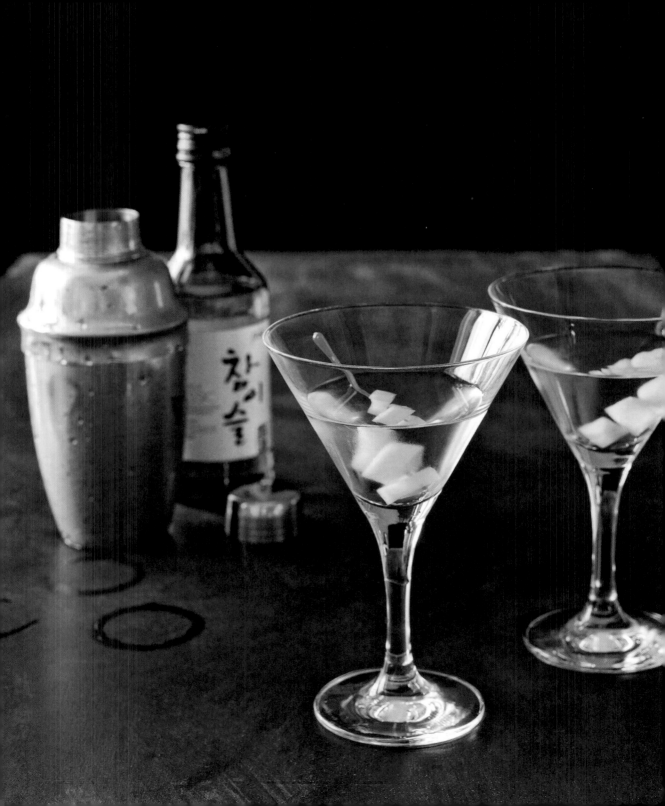

KIMCHITINI

In Korea there is a proverb that goes 'You should not drink the kimchi brine before the kimchi is ready', with the meaning that you should not take things for granted before they happen. However, to enjoy a dry martini with a quirky kimchi twist there is really no need for encouragement.

A Korean type of booze

Soju is sometimes compared to Japanese sake, and in the same way it can be served both warm and cold. Soju could be said to be closer to the spirit category than sake, which is enjoyed more like a wine. Soju is distilled from barley, sweet potato and rice – sometimes a combination of all three and sometimes of just two. The clear spirit often has an alcohol content of 20 per cent. Popular soju bars have started popping up around the world where they serve soju on its own, with lemon juice or in a cocktail.

1. Shake soju, vermouth and ice together in a cocktail shaker.
2. Slice and thread a few pieces of daikon kimchi onto a cocktail stick and place in a martini glass. Pour in the drink. Cheers!

Serves 1

3 tbsp soju or sake
2 tsp dry white vermouth
1 piece rinsed daikon kimchi, see p.28
ice

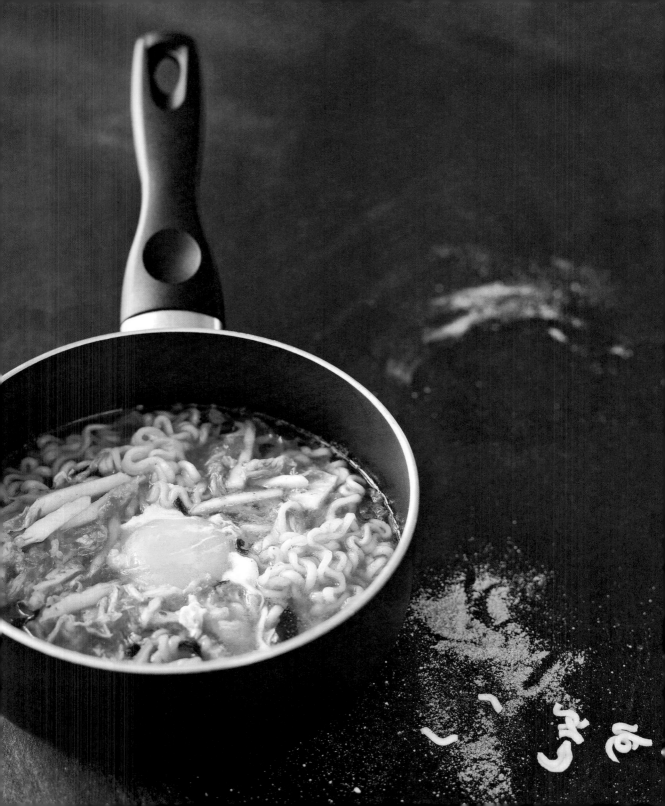

KIMCHI RAMEN

This is 'quick and dirty'. For when you just want something quick or feel like a tasty snack in the evening.

Korean ramen
Koreans eat an abundance of different types of noodles — fresh buckwheat noodles or sweet potato noodles that are stir-fried together with some sesame oil and vegetables. But the cheapest and most immensely popular type is ramen. Ramen is the ultimate student grub, hangover food and snack.

1. Cook the noodles according to the instructions on the package.
2. Crack the egg open and add towards the end of the cooking time and leave it to almost poach. Add the kimchi. Eat!

Serves 1

1 pack (120g/4¼oz) quick noodles
1 egg
30–60g/1–2¼oz/1–2¼oz/¼–½ cup shredded Chinese leaf kimchi (preferably over-fermented), see p.22

HOBAK KIMCHI JJIGAE

SQUASH AND KIMCHI STEW WITH TOFU

Squash kimchi and tofu make the base for a tasty vegetarian stew. But to call it vegetarian in Korea would be a bit strange as no one there would think of a dish as vegetarian or not.

1. Add all the ingredients except the tofu to a pan or casserole dish and simmer, covered with a lid, for about 10 minutes, until the squash is soft but not mushy.
2. Crumble the tofu carefully with your fingers, add to the stew and simmer for a further 5 minutes.
3. Serve with a bowl of boiled rice.

Serves 2-3

225g/8oz/4¼ cups squash kimchi, see p.37
800ml/28fl oz/3⅓ cups water
40g/1½oz/scant ½ cup roughly chopped leek
1 tbsp sesame oil
300g/7oz firm tofu

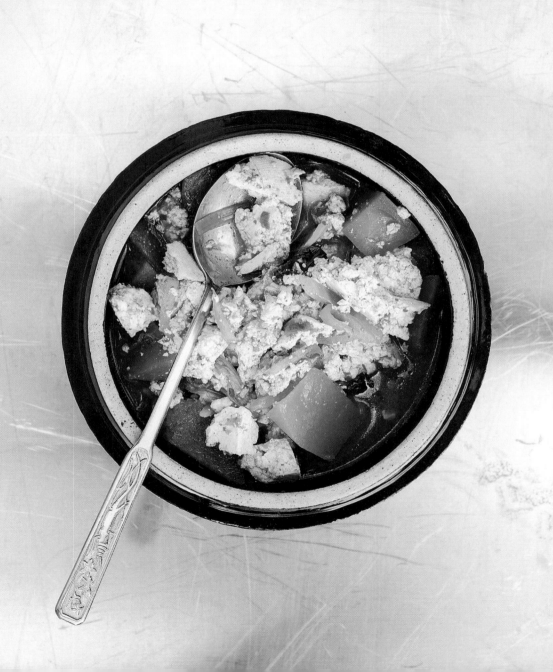

KIMCHI JEON

KIMCHI PANCAKES

In Korea pancakes serve as a cocktail snack or a pleasant side dish. At Arirang it's a popular starter. Easy and quick to make, they go with most things and can be varied infinitely — in this recipe squid and kimchi play the main roles.

1. Boil the squid for 2 minutes and cut it into small pieces.
2. Mix the squid with the other ingredients to form a thick pancake batter.
3. Fry in oil in a frying pan over medium heat. Shape the batter into small pancakes when frying. Cook for a couple of minutes on both sides until the pancakes are golden brown.
4. Mix together all the ingredients for the dipping sauce and serve together with the pancakes.

Serves 2–4

200g/7oz fresh squid
225g/8oz/4¼ cups shredded Chinese leaf kimchi, see p.22
90g/3oz/1 cup finely chopped leek
225g/8oz/heaped 1¾ cups plain flour
1 egg
1 tbsp sesame oil
cooking oil for frying

Dipping sauce
4 tbsp Korean or Japanese soy sauce
1 dash distilled vinegar, 12%
½ tbsp sesame oil
1 tbsp finely shredded spring onion

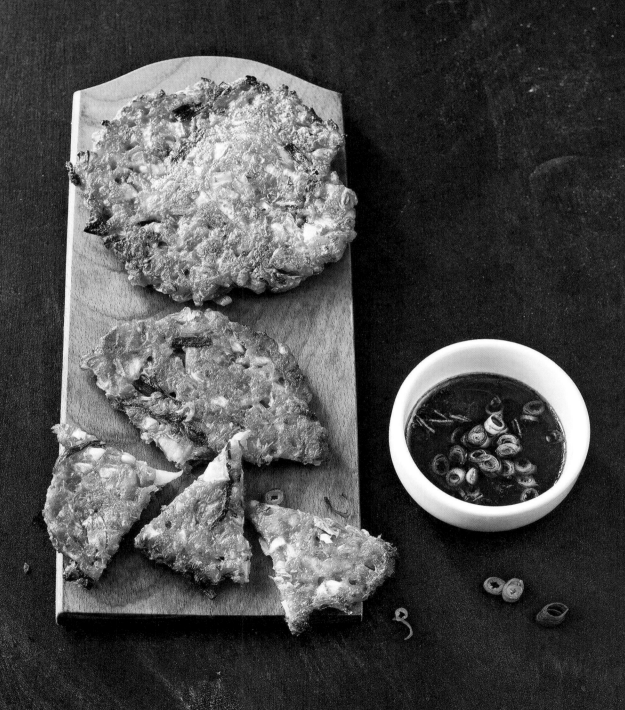

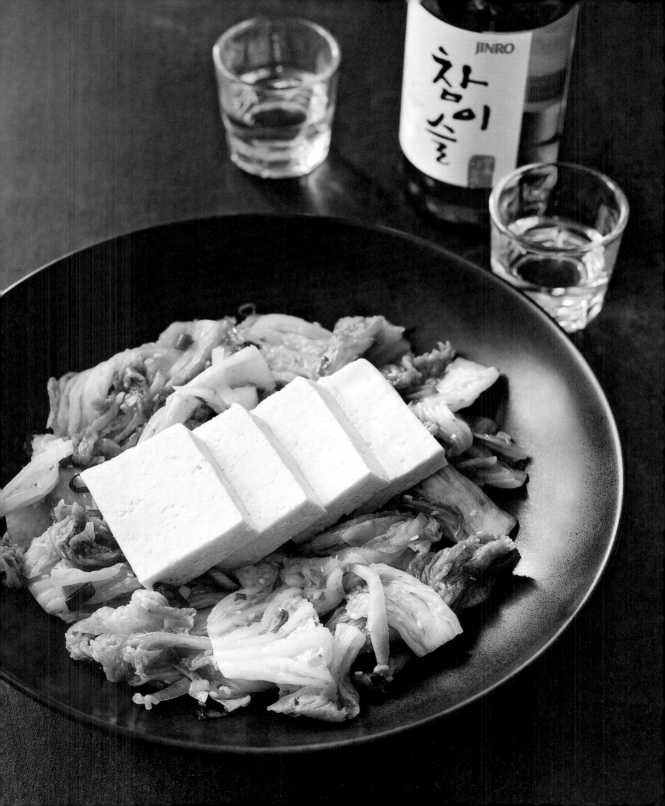

TOBU KIMCHI

TOFU KIMCHI

There are a lot of variations of this dish. Here the tofu is poached, but you can also fry it. If you make a version that is not very spicy it will be nice as a cocktail snack.

Different kinds of tofu

Tofu is made from soya beans and is popular in large parts of Asia. There are different kinds of tofu that go together with different types of dishes. For the tobu kimchi on this page you will need a hard and firm tofu that will stay together and not break. The soft and smooth silken tofu is, for example, used for the popular stew sundubu jjigae.

1. Slice the tofu into large cubes or even larger domino tiles.
2. Poach the tofu for 2 minutes and plate up on a dish together with the kimchi. Drizzle over the sesame oil and sprinkle with some sesame seeds.

Serves 2–4

Approx. 400g/14oz firm tofu
150g/5oz/1¼ cups shredded Chinese leaf kimchi, see p.22
2 tbsp sesame oil
toasted sesame seeds

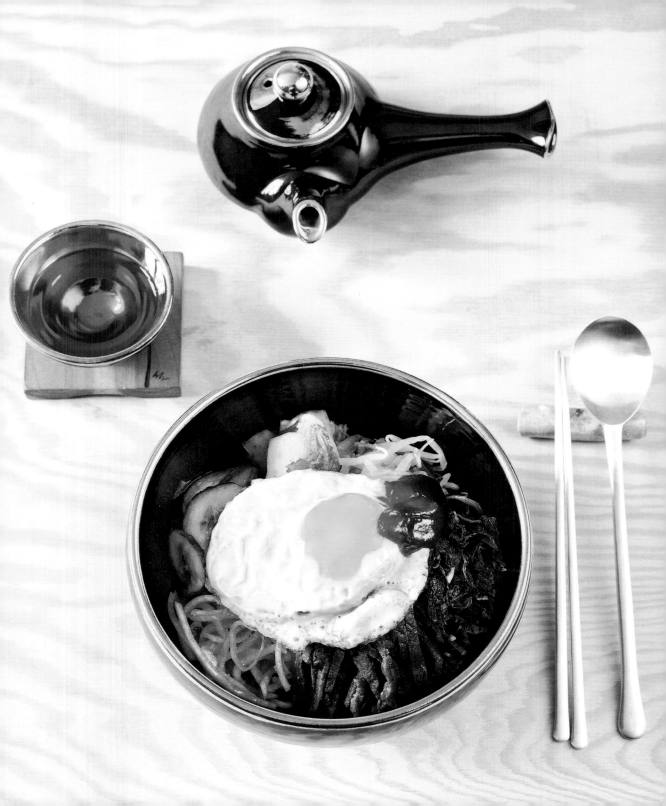

BIBIMBAP

Bibimbap is Arirang's – as well as Korea's – signature dish. Traditionally it is a rice dish that is garnished with different marinated vegetables, meat and egg. When you eat *bibimbap* you take a dollop of chilli paste and mix it together with all the ingredients using a spoon. It's useful to make big batches of the vegetables while you are at it; they are superb as sides for most Korean dishes.

In Korea there are different kinds of regional versions of bibimbap; perhaps we should name ours 'Stockholm bibimbap'. Even visiting Koreans think it is tastier than in Korea.

1. Rinse the rice repeatedly in cold water until the water comes out almost completely clear. Boil in a rice cooker or a pan. If you are using a pan: bring to boil at high heat. When the lid starts moving, turn down to medium heat. Simmer for 10 minutes. Turn down to the lowest heat setting and simmer for a further 10 minutes. Leave to rest covered with a lid for 10 minutes before serving. Never use salt when boiling rice.
2. Prepare the different marinated vegetables and fry the bulgogi according to the directions for each recipe.
3. Fry the eggs.
4. Construct the *bibimbap*: first put cooked rice in the bottom of four serving bowls, top with grilled meat and the marinated vegetables. Finish off by placing the fried egg on top. Serve with a small bowl of chilli paste on the side so that everyone can add as much as they wish.

Serves 4

320g/11¼oz/heaped 1⅔ cups short-grain rice
40g/1½oz/⅓ cup sesame-marinated bean sprouts, see p.94
40g/1½oz/⅓ cup spice-marinated cucumber, see p.94
225g/8oz/scant 3¾ cups kimchi of your choice
100g/3¼oz/½ cup marinated spinach, see p.94
100g/3¼oz/1 cup marinated daikon, see p.94
220g/7¼oz/2 cups bulgogi, see p.106
4 eggs
Approx. 30g/1oz/½ cup *gochujang*, Korean chilli paste

KIMCHI IN FOOD

OI NAMUL SPICE-MARINATED CUCUMBER

1. Finely slice the cucumber.
2. Mix together all the ingredients for the marinade. Add the cucumber and leave to marinate for 30 minutes.

1 cucumber

Marinade
20g/¾oz/½ cup finely chopped leek
½ tbsp granulated sugar
1 tsp rice vinegar
1 tsp salt
1 tsp *gochugaru*, Korean chilli powder

SOOKJU NAMUL SESAME-MARINATED BEAN SPROUTS

1. Clean and trim the bean sprouts before quickly parboiling them in boiling water. Rinse in cold water a few times. Drain and mix the sprouts together with salt and sesame oil.

40g/1½oz/scant ½ cup fresh bean sprouts
1 tsp salt
1 tsp sesame oil

SHIGUMCHI NAMUL MARINATED SPINACH

1. Parboil the spinach quickly in boiling water. Rinse in cold water a few times and squeeze the water out with your hands. Cut it into thinner slices and marinate with salt, leek and sesame oil.

200g/7oz fresh baby spinach
½ tbsp salt
2 tbsp finely chopped leek
1 tbsp sesame oil

MOO NAMUL MARINATED DAIKON

1. Peel and shred the daikon. Boil in a pan over medium heat for 5–10 minutes until it's slightly transparent.
2. Drain off the water but leave the daikon in the pan. Add the other ingredients and warm through quickly. Can be eaten both lukewarm and cold.

350g/12oz fresh daikon (mooli)
40g/1½oz/scant ½ cup finely shredded leek
1 tbsp sesame oil
1 pinch minced garlic
½ tbsp salt

KONG JANG MARINATED SOYA BEANS

1. Rinse the soya beans. Place them in a pan and add water to just cover the beans. Leave to stand for 2–3 hours, until the beans have soaked up some water.
2. Place the pan on the stove and bring to the boil. When the water has almost evaporated, add soy sauce and sugar and simmer on a low heat for 30 minutes whilst stirring, until the beans feel soft enough. Will keep for 2–3 months in the fridge.

500g/1lb 2oz dried black soya beans
100ml/3½fl oz/scant ½ cup Korean or Japanese soy sauce
75g/2¾oz/scant ½ cup granulated sugar

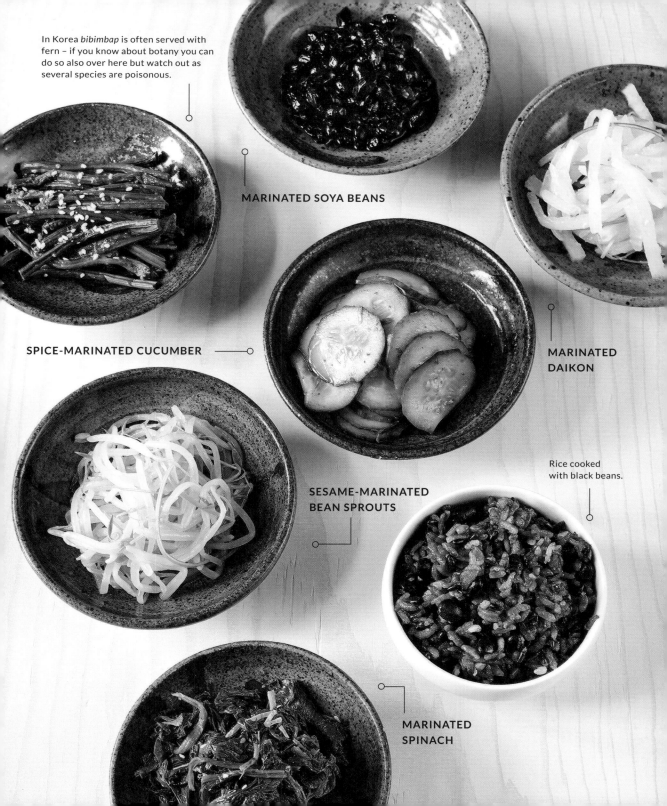

In Korea *bibimbap* is often served with fern – if you know about botany you can do so also over here but watch out as several species are poisonous.

MARINATED SOYA BEANS

SPICE-MARINATED CUCUMBER

MARINATED DAIKON

SESAME-MARINATED
BEAN SPROUTS

Rice cooked
with black beans.

MARINATED SPINACH

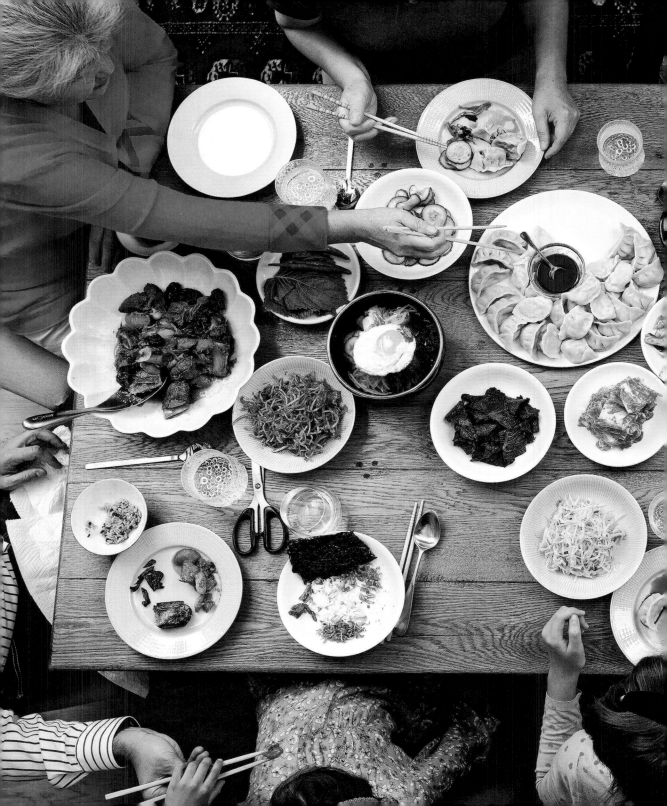

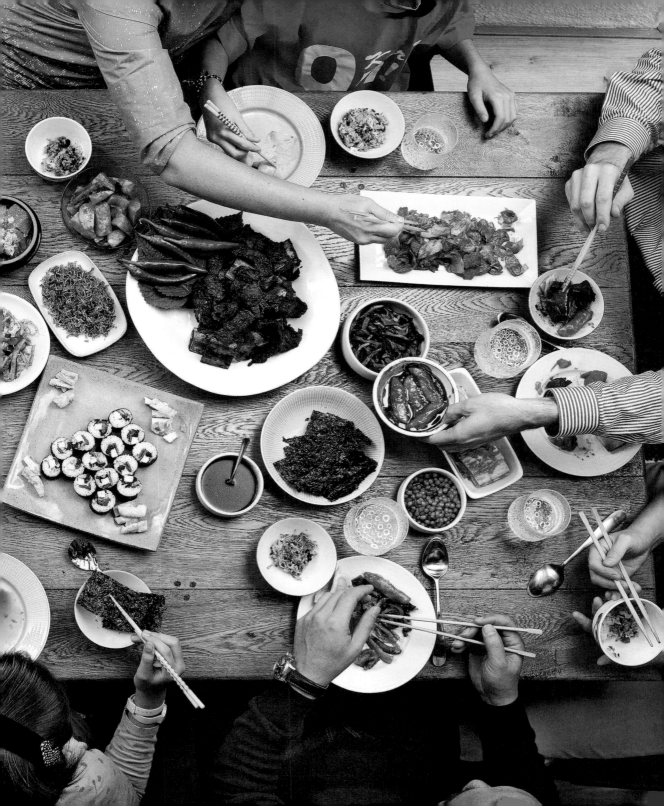

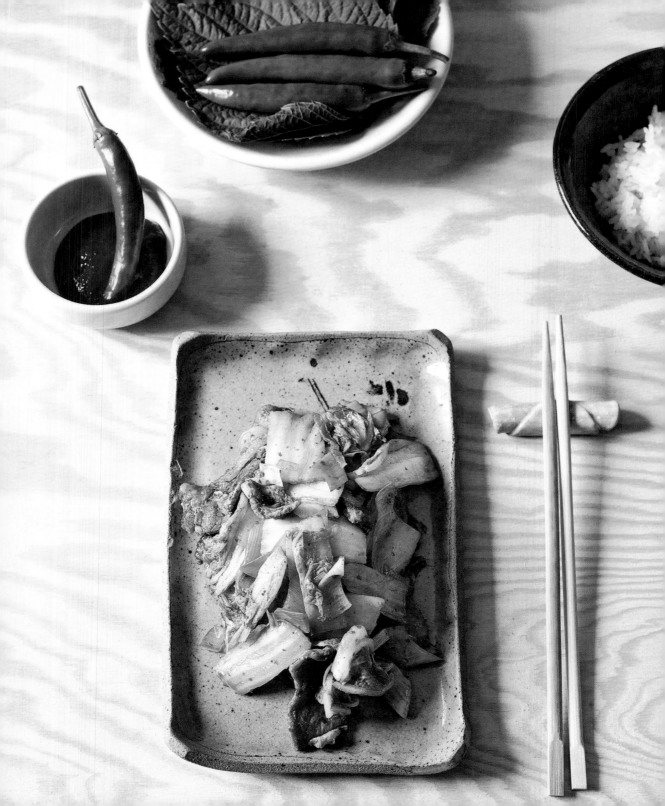

KIMCHI BOKKUM

FRIED KIMCHI WITH PORK

A kimchi that has matured for some time is the best option for this dish. The dish requires the meat to be properly fried and not boiled. If you are cooking for several people you will therefore have to fry the meat in batches. If you want to eat vegetarian you can swap the meat for tofu. *Bokkum* means 'to fry', and often the rice is also fried. Specialised *Bokkum* restaurants in Korea offer endless varieties of this typical comfort food — but it works just as well at home.

1. Slice the pork collar thinly and fry in oil in a hot frying pan until golden.
2. Add the kimchi and the leek and fry for another 5 minutes.
3. Add the sugar and the sesame oil and fry for another minute. Serve with boiled rice.

Serves 1–2

200g/7oz pork collar or pork belly
225g/8oz/scant 3¾ cups Chinese leaf kimchi, see p.22
90g/3oz/1 cup shredded leek
½ tbsp granulated sugar
1 tbsp sesame oil
cooking oil for frying

OYSTER DRESSING

This is a fun variation of the standard vinaigrette that is served with oysters. Traditionally, leftover kimchi brine is not used, but it feels wasteful not to do anything with it — and the oysters will get a real kick to them.

1. Finely chop the daikon kimchi into tiny little pieces.
2. Mix the brine with the daikon. Add sugar to taste. Serve with newly opened oysters and some finely shredded cucumber (optional).

30g/1oz/⅔ cup daikon kimchi, see p.28
4 tbsp kimchi brine
1 pinch sugar (if needed)

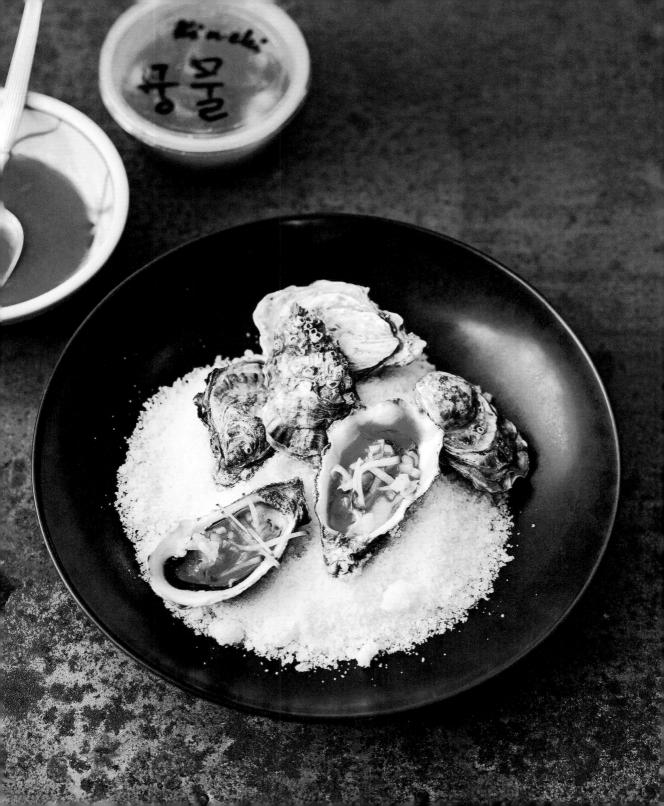

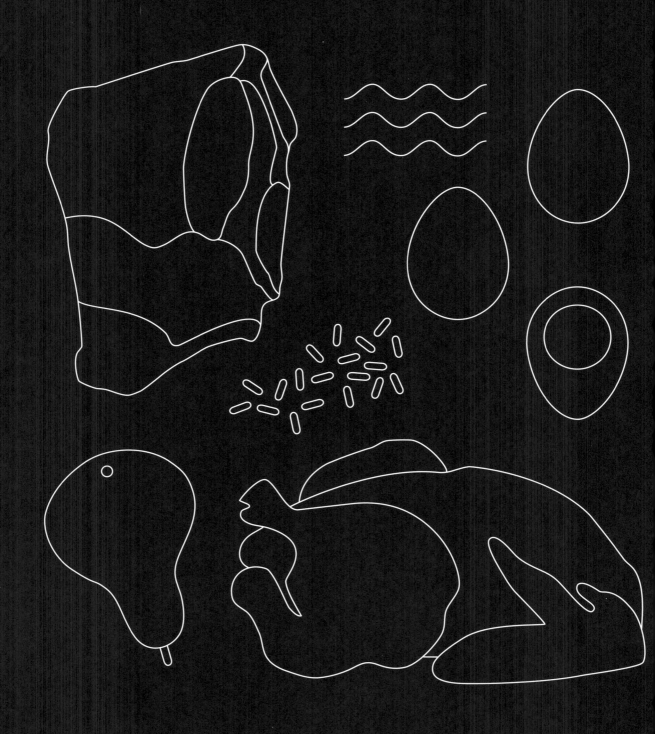

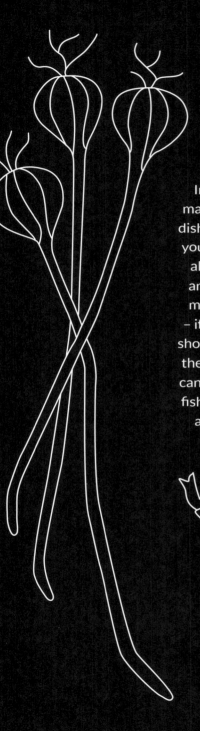

OTHER KOREAN DISHES

In Korea, a meal isn't made up of starter, main and dessert – instead a lot of different dishes and sides are put out on the table, and you enjoy them together. A social meal, that also allows you to show your compassion and care for your near and dear ones. The meal can even become a way to apologise – if you've had a row with someone you can show your regret by, for example, dishing out the best bits for that person. A Korean meal can contain different soups, stews, meat and fish dishes, salads and sides, but one thing is always present on the table: the kimchi.

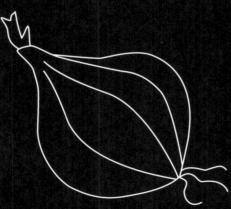

The perfect spoon has a long, thin handle and a shallow bowl with a smooth edge to fit the mouth better.

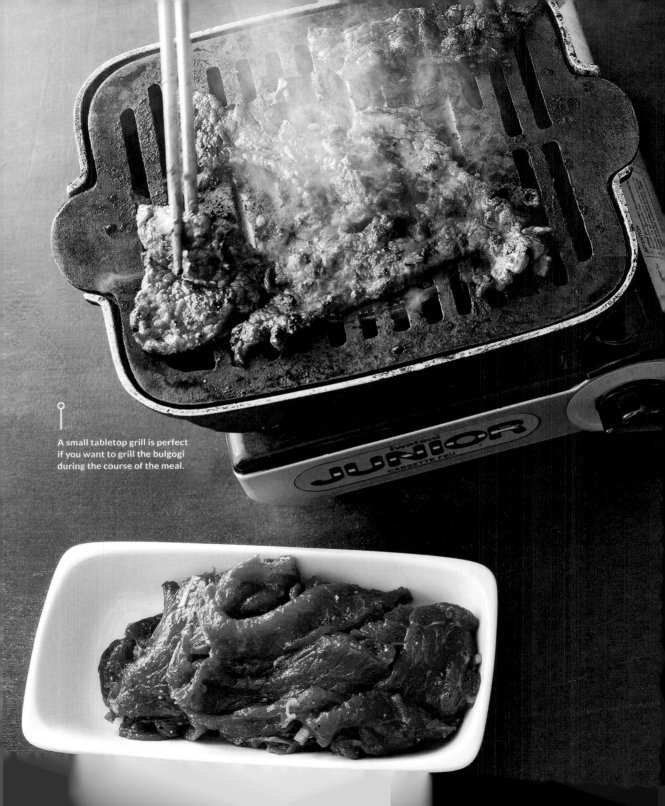

A small tabletop grill is perfect if you want to grill the bulgogi during the course of the meal.

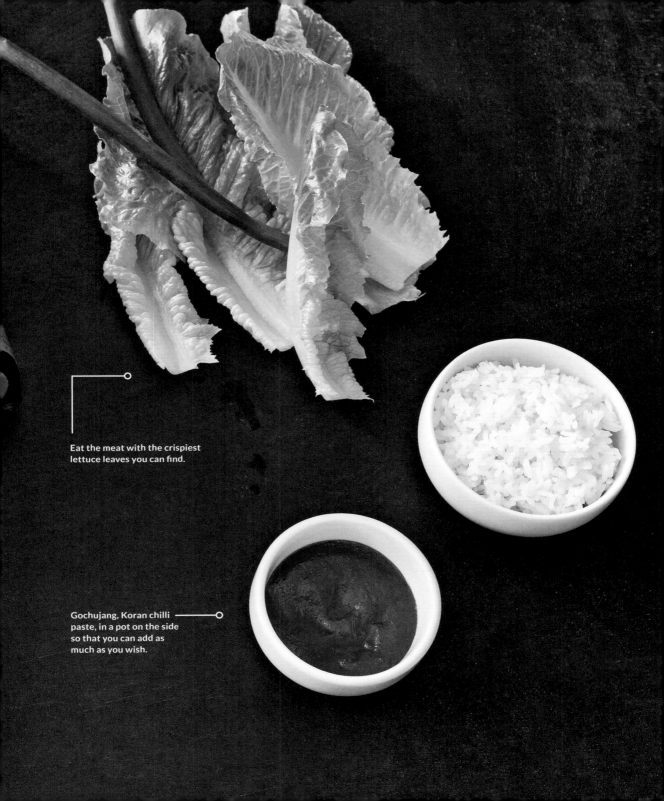

Eat the meat with the crispiest lettuce leaves you can find.

Gochujang, Koran chilli paste, in a pot on the side so that you can add as much as you wish.

BULGOGI

MARINATED BEEF

In Korea, almost all households have a small tabletop grill — either a gas or an electric one. **Everyone** loves to grill and **no one** is put off by the cooking fumes.

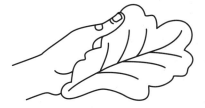

Place a salad leaf in your hand.

Serves 4–6

800g/1lb 12oz beef sirloin, tenderloin, skirt or rib eye steak

Marinade
1 tbsp minced garlic
1½ tbsp sesame oil
100ml/3½fl oz/scant ½ cup Korean or Japanese soy sauce
2 tbsp granulated sugar
½ pinch black pepper

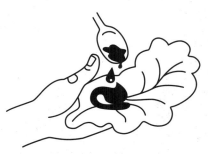

Add a dollop of *gochujang*.

1. Place the meat in the freezer for a while to make it easier to cut into thin slices, about 3–4cm/1¼–1½in thick. You could also ask for thin slices at the butcher's.
2. Mix together all the ingredients for the marinade and add the meat. Marinate for 30 minutes in the fridge.
3. Grill or fry the meat on a high heat. As the slices are thin they cook very quickly.
4. Dig in! Serve the meat with salad, rice, kimchi, different side dishes and chilli paste.

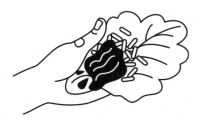

Add some rice on top and finish off with meat.

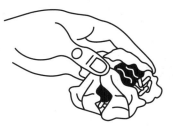

Fold the leaf into a parcel and eat!

OTHER KOREAN DISHES

SAMGYEOPSAL

GRILLED PORK BELLY

SAMGYEOPSAL-GUI

MARINATED PORK BELLY

Pure pork flavour with sesame oil. It's the fat the gives the meat its flavour. Remember to use fresh and not cured pork belly. Of course, kimchi goes perfectly well with this.

Grilled pork belly is super tasty to eat together with a salad leaf. Add some extra chilli paste to the leaf if you like your food a bit hotter. It's good to prepare enough meat to have some leftover, which is perfect in a baguette (see p.110).

Serves 2–3

400g/14oz uncured pork belly, sliced

Sesame salt
3½ tbsp sesame oil
1 tbsp salt
1 pinch black pepper

1. Mix sesame oil, salt and pepper in a small bowl.
2. Grill the pork belly on a hot stove-top grill pan for 15–20 minutes, or you can cook it in the oven at 200°C/400°F/Gas Mark 6, or fry in a pan on medium heat.
3. Dip the grilled meat in the sesame salt and eat together with rice and kimchi.

Serves 4–6

800g/1lb 12oz uncured pork belly, sliced

Marinade
4 tbsp *gochujang*, Korean chilli paste
2 tbsp minced garlic
1 tbsp grated ginger
4 tbsp granulated sugar
1 tsp black pepper
2 tbsp sesame oil

1. Pre-heat the oven to 200°C/400°F/Gas Mark 6.
2. Mix together all the ingredients for the marinade. Fold in the pork belly and mix thoroughly.
3. Arrange the pork slices on a hot stove-top grill pan or in a deep pan suitable for the oven. The slices should not overlap each other.
4. Grill or cook in the middle of the oven for 15–20 minutes, until the meat is golden brown and crispy. Flip the slices over once or twice during the cooking. Serve with a bowl of rice and preferably salad leaves and some marinated vegetables.

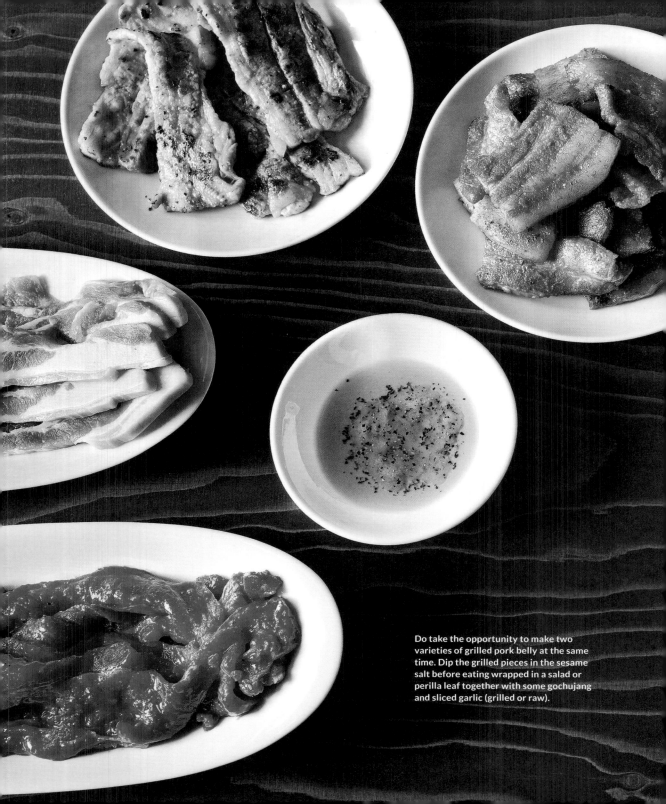

Do take the opportunity to make two varieties of grilled pork belly at the same time. Dip the grilled pieces in the sesame salt before eating wrapped in a salad or perilla leaf together with some gochujang and sliced garlic (grilled or raw).

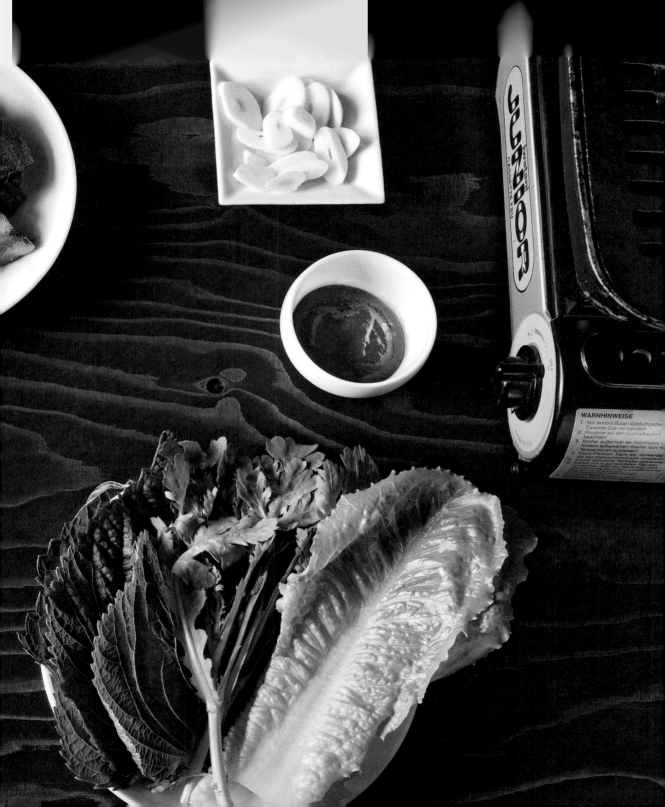

BAGUETTE WITH BULGOGI OR SAMGYEOPSAL

This is the staff breakfast at the restaurant.
A baguette from the neighbouring bakery,
filled with any of the side dishes. Egg makes
everything delicious. You should never underrate
a tasty sandwich.

1. Slice the baguette into four parts. Cut them open lengthwise.
2. Fill with meat, vegetables and egg. Eat!

Serves 4

1 baguette
200g/7oz bulgogi or samgyeopsal, see p.106 or p.107
300g/10½oz sesame-marinated bean sprouts, see p.94
4 fried eggs
120g/4¼oz/1¼ cups Chinese leaf kimchi, see p.22
kimchi butter, see p.74, or *gochujang*, Korean chilli paste

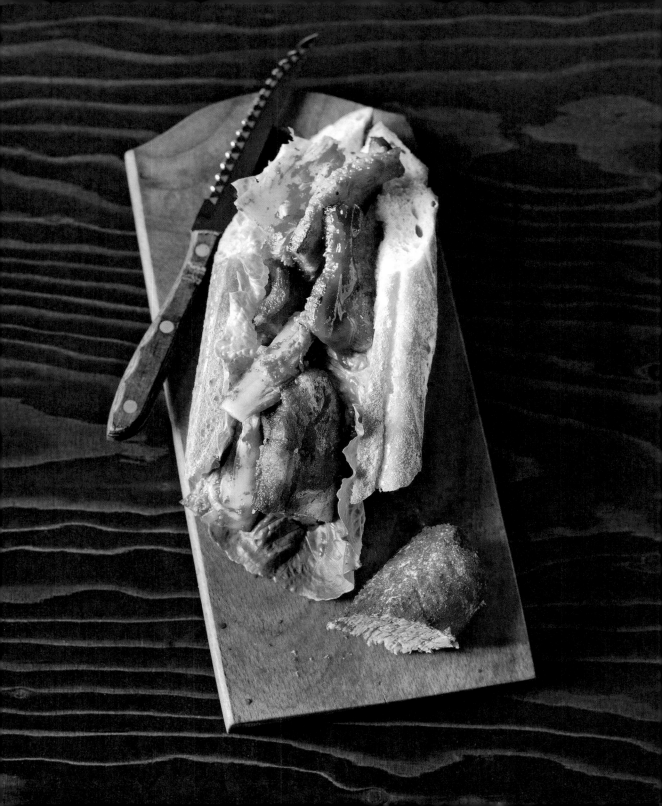

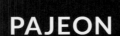

PAJEON

KOREAN PANCAKES WITH SPRING ONION

A super tasty starter. Child-friendly but also well suited as a cocktail snack or together with a cold lager. In Korea it's a popular street food, you'll recognise the pancake from the spring onions.

Bar snacks

Koreans are very fond of bar snacks. If you're out drinking in any of the traditional places (there are both Korean and Western bars in Korea) you'll often find you can't just have a drink but will have to order a snack too, such as the popular pancake varieties pajeon *and* bindaetteok.

1. Mix together the ingredients for the dipping sauce and leave to one side.
2. Slice the green stems of the spring onions into 3–4cm/1¼–1½in long pieces, discard the white bulbs. Mix together flour, water, garlic, salt and pepper to a thick, smooth batter. Add the onions.
3. Fry the batter in batches like pancakes, approx. 5mm/¼in thick, in a little oil in a frying pan on medium heat for 3–5 minutes, until golden brown on both sides.
4. Serve with the dipping sauce.

1 bunch spring onions
85g/2¾oz/⅔ cup plain flour
4 tbsp water
1 garlic clove
salt and black pepper
cooking oil for frying

Soy dipping sauce
4 tbsp Korean or Japanese soy sauce
1 dash distilled vinegar, 12%

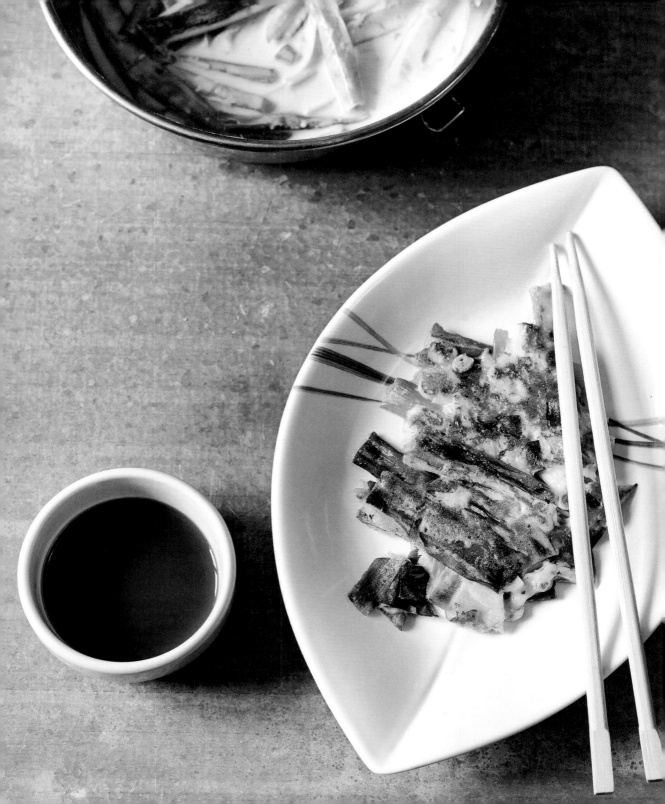

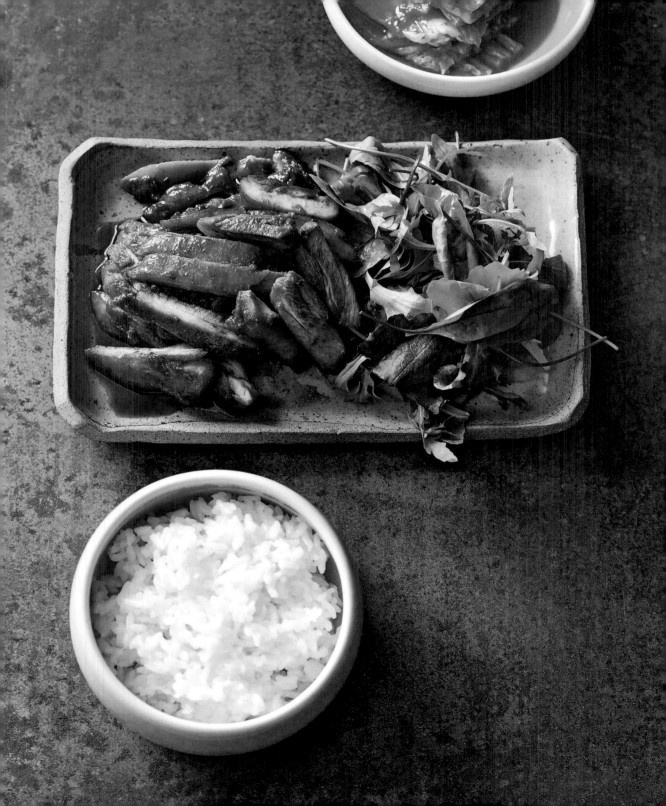

DAK GALBI

MARINATED CHICKEN THIGHS

There are plenty of different family recipes for this much-loved dish – this is Arirang's version. However, once you've tried it, make your own version – there are no directives or rules. The dish has been developed as a slightly cheaper alternative to the festive dish *so galbi*, where beef brisket is grilled instead of chicken. In Korea there are places that specialise in *dak galbi* where they serve high-quality chicken marinated in a hot sauce and then grilled on large griddles.

1. Rinse the chicken and pat it dry. Slice into smaller pieces.
2. Mix together all the ingredients for the marinade, add the chicken and leave to marinate for about 15 minutes.
3. Take the chicken out of the marinade and fry in oil in a frying pan on medium heat for 10–15 minutes until cooked through.
4. Serve with boiled rice, salad leaves and kimchi.

Serves 4

600g/1lb 5oz chicken thigh fillets
cooking oil for frying

Marinade
4 tbsp ketchup
4 tbsp *chunjang*, black soya bean paste
2 tbsp *gochujang*, Korean chilli paste
4 tbsp Korean or Japanese soy sauce
½ tbsp minced garlic
½ tbsp grated ginger
1 tbsp granulated sugar
2 tbsp sesame oil

OTHER KOREAN DISHES

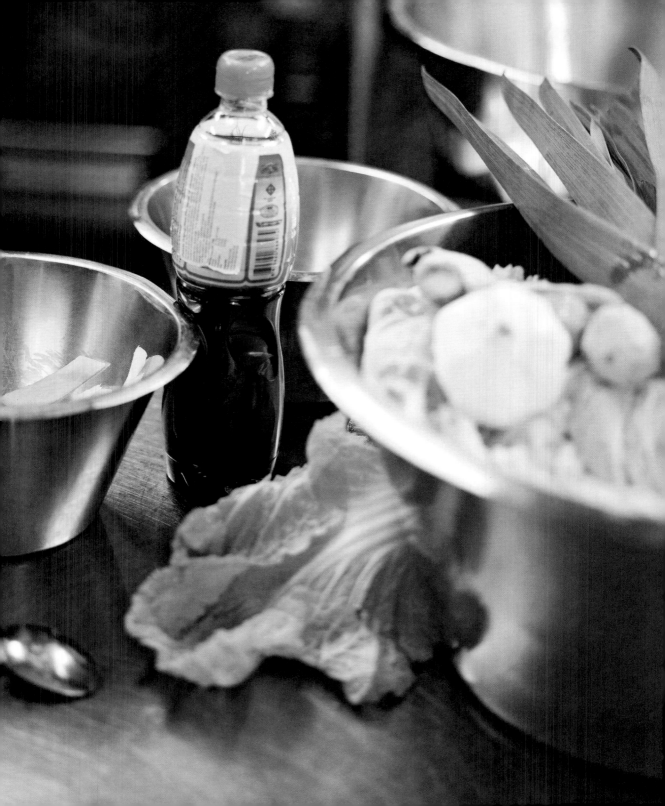

<u>삼계탕</u>
  찹쌀 마늘 후추가루 소금 대추
  닭 찹쌀.

<u>된장 찌개 med kimchi</u>
파. 두부. 소금. 후추가루. 감자 마늘?

<u>꽃게장 (Small kimchi)</u>
깨후. 고추가루. 마늘. 파. 오이
참기름 깨 넣은 쌀눈

— 감자 쉽쓰 만드르나나 —

간장마늘

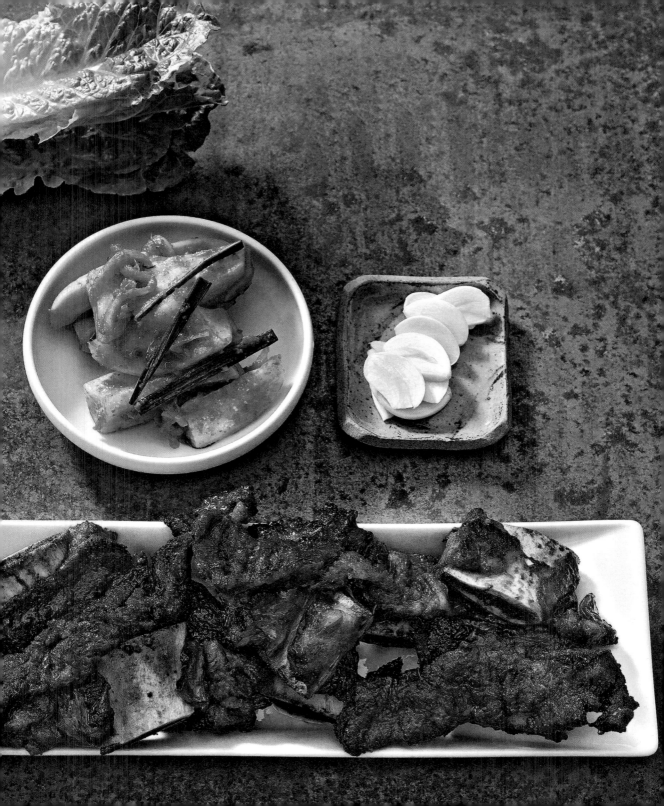

SO GALBI

MARINATED BRISKET

Beef brisket is a favourite meat among Koreans — a delicacy that takes time to prepare! It's the meat and the connective tissue nearest to the bone that are the tasty bits so you'll have to get chewing. The pear is added as it's said to tenderise the meat.

'When Byung-Soon's children were little they got brisket bones to chew on instead of plastic teething rings. We think it's great to learn to gnaw at an early age; it's just like proper eating.'

1. Buy a brisket on the bone that is cut against the meat fibres into 5cm/1¼in-thick slices. Slice the meat according to the instructions on p.120.
2. Peel and finely chop pear and onion. Mix together with the other ingredients for the marinade.
3. Pour the marinade over the brisket and mix thoroughly. Leave to marinate for 30 minutes in the fridge.
4. Fry the meat in a hot frying pan for approx. 15 minutes (alternatively grill on a table-top grill or in the oven at 200°C/400°F/Gas Mark 6). Serve with boiled rice, salad leaves, sliced garlic and preferably some side dishes.

1kg/2lb 4oz beef brisket
cooking oil for frying (if needed)

Marinade
1 pear
½ brown onion
90g/3oz/1 cup chopped leek
1 tbsp minced garlic
100ml/3½fl oz/scant ½ cup Korean or Japanese
    soy sauce
75g/2½oz/scant ½ cup granulated sugar
1 tsp black pepper
4 tbsp sesame oil

GALBI

Brisket can be tough. When you slice it like this, it becomes easier to marinate and tenderise the meat.

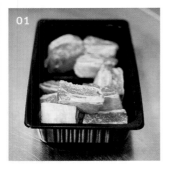

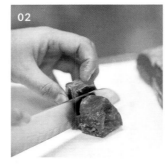

01. Buy brisket on the bone that is cut against the meat fibres into 5cm/2in-thick slices.

02–03. Cut along the bone almost all the way through, leave about 5mm/¼in.

04–07. Cut the meat carefully at the same time as you roll it out so that you get a long thin strip that is still attached to the bone at one edge. Almost like the movement you use when you're spreading butter.

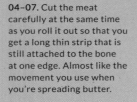

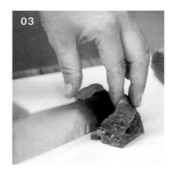

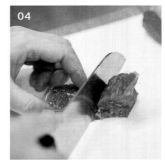

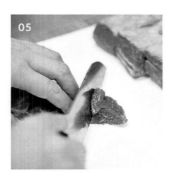

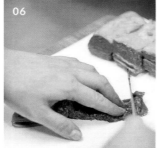

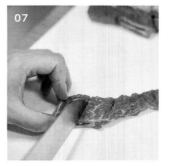

OTHER KOREAN DISHES

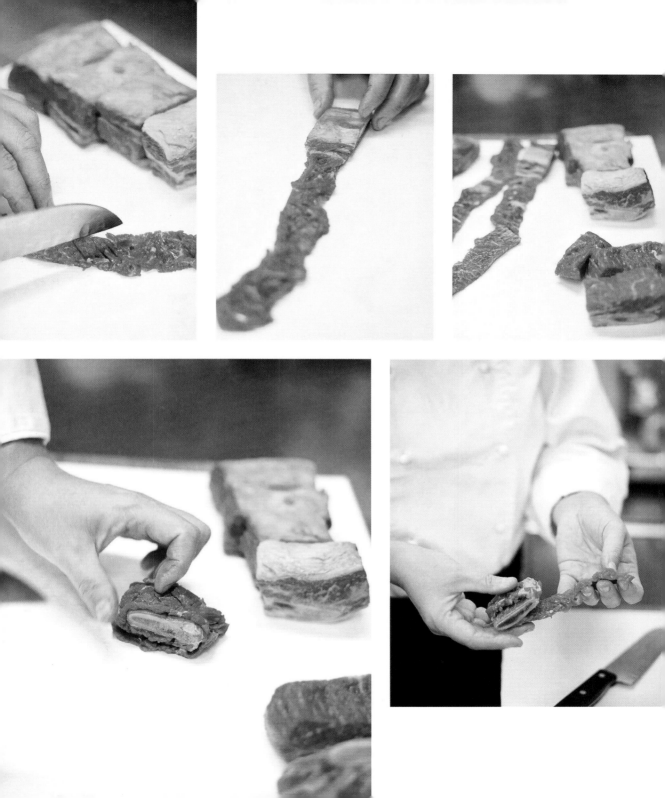

YUKGAEJANG

HOT BEEF CHUCK SOUP

A warming soup made from beef chuck. Goes well together with some *namul* sides, for example marinated spinach (see p.94).

1. Place the rib in a pan and cover with water. Bring to the boil and leave to simmer covered with a lid for about one hour.
2. Mix together all the ingredients for the chilli paste in a bowl.
3. Leave the meat to cool and then tear it into strips using your fingers. Slice spring onion and Chinese leaf.
4. Skim off the fat from the stock and reheat. Add a stock cube if you wish, add the vegetables and simmer for a few minutes on medium heat.
5. Mix all but 1 tbsp of the chilli paste with the meat.
6. Add the reserved 1 tbsp of chilli paste to the simmering stock.
7. Finish off by adding the meat to the stock and simmer for a few more minutes. Serve with a bowl of boiled rice.

Serves 3–4

80g/2¾oz/heaped ¾ cup fresh bean sprouts
2 bunches spring onions
1 Chinese leaf, the green part
500g/1lb 2oz beef chuck
1 beef stock cube (optional)

Chilli paste
2 tbsp *gochugaru*, Korean chilli powder
1 tbsp *gochujang*, Korean chilli paste
1 tbsp minced garlic
½ tbsp grated ginger
1 tsp black pepper
½ tsp salt

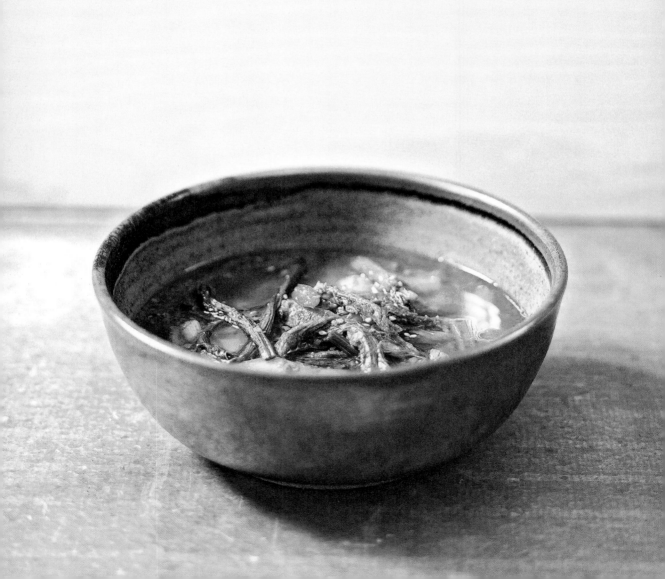

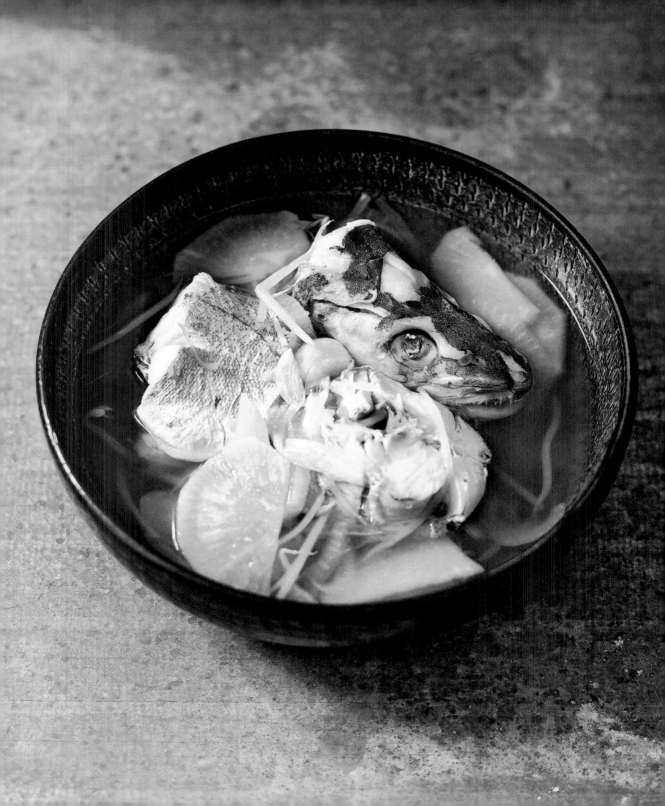

SAENGSON JJIGAE

FISH SOUP

In Korea the whole fish is used for making soup to ensure the broth is as tasty as possible. But on the other hand, you wouldn't serve the head to guests.

1. Peel and slice the onion.
2. Add all the ingredients to a wide pan or casserole dish and cover with water. Bring to the boil and simmer gently for approx. 5 minutes, until the vegetables are almost cooked through. Add the fish and simmer covered with a lid for about 10 minutes.
3. Add salt and pepper to taste. Serve with a bowl of boiled rice.

Serves 3–4

1 whole whiting (approx. 500g/1lb 2oz) or other firm white fish
1 brown onion
100g/3½oz/1 cup sliced fresh daikon (mooli)
100g/3½oz/1 cup coarsely sliced leek
100g/3½oz/1 cup fresh bean sprouts
1 tbsp finely grated ginger
½ tbsp finely chopped garlic
salt and black pepper

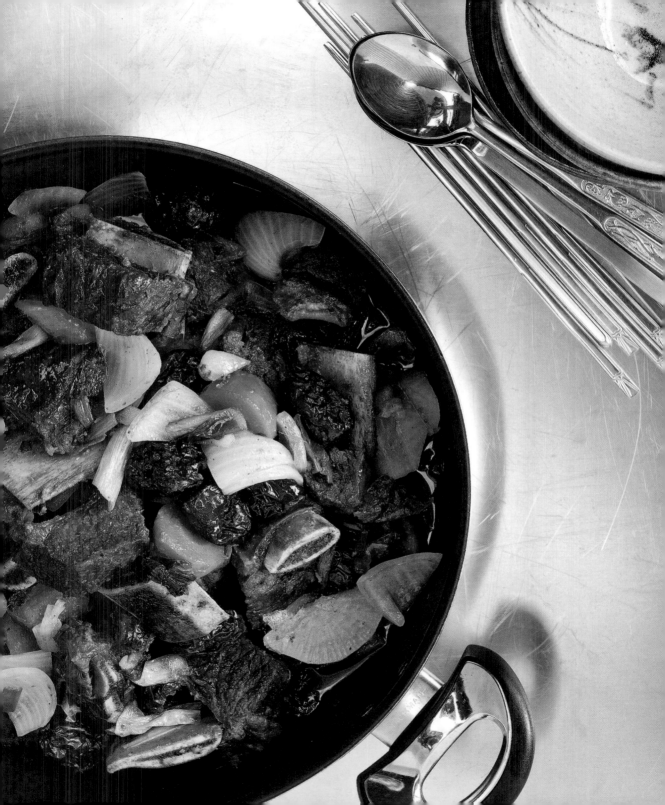

GALBI JJIM

BRISKET STEW

Slightly complicated to prepare, but worth all
the effort. A large batch is perfect for freezing.
You can leave out the jujube fruits, but they
are available to buy in most Asian food stores.
If you can't get hold of brisket you can use
chuck – perhaps cut a large bit in two and make
yukgaejang (p.122) the day after?

1. Rinse the brisket in cold water and slice the
   meat in between the ribs into stewing pieces.
2. Place the meat in a casserole dish or a pan and
   cover with water. Bring to the boil and discard
   the water. Cover with fresh water and simmer
   for approx. 30 minutes.
3. Mix together all the ingredients for the
   marinade.
4. Take the meat out of the pan, but keep the
   stock. Place the meat in a separate bowl
   together with the marinade and leave to
   marinate for 15 minutes.
5. Peel and chop daikon, carrot and leek into
   approx. 3cm/1¼in large cubes.
6. Add daikon, carrot and jujube fruits to the
   stock that's left in the pan from cooking the
   meat. Simmer for approx. 20 minutes.
7. Add the marinated meat to the stew together
   with onion and leek. Simmer for about
   10 minutes, until the stew has reduced a little.

1kg/2lb 4oz beef brisket
400g/14oz fresh daikon (mooli)
300g/10½oz carrot
2 brown onions
½ leek
10 jujube fruits (optional)
a few fresh chestnuts

Marinade
100ml/3½fl oz/scant ½ cup Korean or Japanese
   soy sauce
45g/1½oz/¼ cup granulated sugar
2 tbsp golden syrup
45g/1½oz/scant ½ cup finely chopped leek
2 tbsp minced garlic
2 tbsp sesame oil

OTHER KOREAN DISHES

NAENG MYEON

NOODLES IN CHILLED BROTH

Naeng means chilled and *myeon* means noodles. In all Asian countries cold noodles are eaten during the summer. This is a popular dish in Korea. You can make a simpler version by using the brine from the winter kimchi (see p.46) instead of stock. If you want it really cold, just add some ice cubes to the broth.

Korean noodles

Korans really love their noodles. The noodles are named depending on what they're made from, if they're long or short, flat or round. There are three main categories: wheat noodles, mil myeon, *that are found in ramen soup, for example; buckwheat noodles,* memil myeon, *that are used foremost for chilled noodle dishes like* naeng myeon *and* bibim myeon; *and finally sweet potato noodles like* dangmyeon, *which makes the base for* japchae.

1. Place the chuck in a pan and cover with water. Simmer for 30 minutes. Leave to cool and slice thinly.
2. Prepare the broth in a separate pan by bringing water to the boil and adding the stock cubes. It should be somewhat under-seasoned. Leave to cool and skim off any fat. Add sugar and distilled vinegar to taste.
3. Cook the noodles according to the instructions on the package. Rinse a few times in cold water.
4. Halve the eggs, shred the cucumber and peel and shred the pear.
5. Pour the broth into soup bowls, add the noodles and top with cucumber, pear, kimchi and egg halves. Serve with a dollop of mustard on the side.

Serves 2

150g/5oz beef chuck, diced
250g/9oz *naengmyeon* noodles,
    Korean buckwheat noodles
2 boiled eggs
½ cucumber
1 pear
Approx. 100g/3¾oz/1 cup white kimchi, see p.31,
    winter kimchi, see p.46 or
    rinsed Chinese leaf kimchi, see p.22
Approx. 1 tbsp Dijon mustard

Noodle broth

1.5 litres/2½ pints/16½ cups water
2 beef stock cubes
Approx. 1 tbsp granulated sugar
Approx. 1 tbsp distilled vinegar, 12%

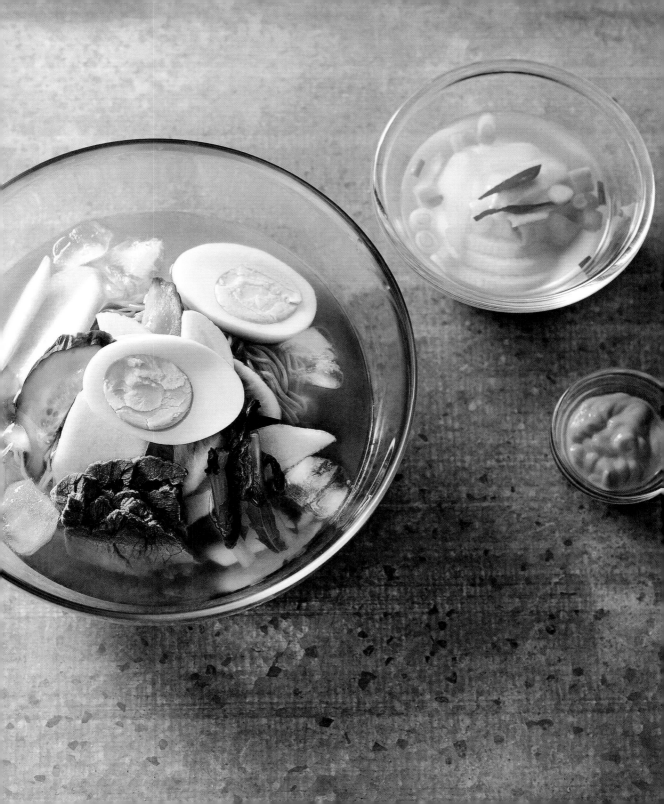

BIBIM MYEON

HOT CHILLED NOODLES

This is one of the most popular Korean summer dishes. If you have any leftover pickled vegetables from making, for example, *bibimbap*, just chuck them in here together with some shredded cucumber. Although for this recipe in particular you don't have to parboil the vegetables, it works fine with cold, crispy veg – just as if you were making a noodle salad. Normally rice isn't served together with noodles, except for *japchae*, which is often served as a side dish.

1. Finely shred the pear and slice the cucumber. Boil and peel the eggs and cut them in half.
2. Cook the noodles according to the instructions on the package.
3. Mix together all the ingredients except for the eggs and stir thoroughly. Finish off by placing the eggs on top and garnish with some extra sesame seeds.

Serves 2

1 pear
½ cucumber
2 eggs
Approx. 250g/9oz *naengmyeon* noodles, Korean buckwheat noodles
3 tbsp *gochujang*, Korean chilli paste
1 tsp distilled vinegar, 12%
2 tbsp granulated sugar
1 tbsp sesame oil
1 tbsp chopped leek
1 tsp minced garlic
1 tsp toasted sesame seeds
50–100g/1¾–3½oz/½–1 cup finely sliced kimchi of your choice

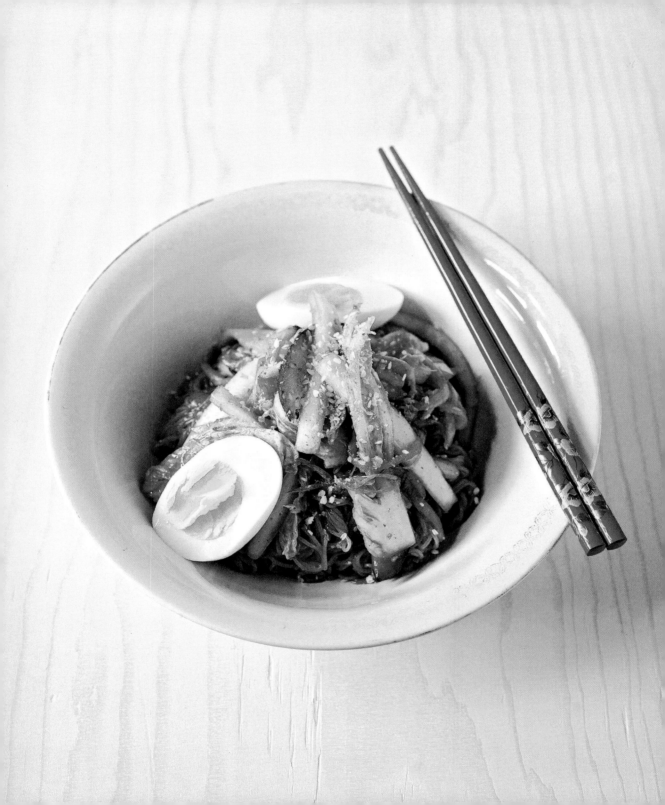

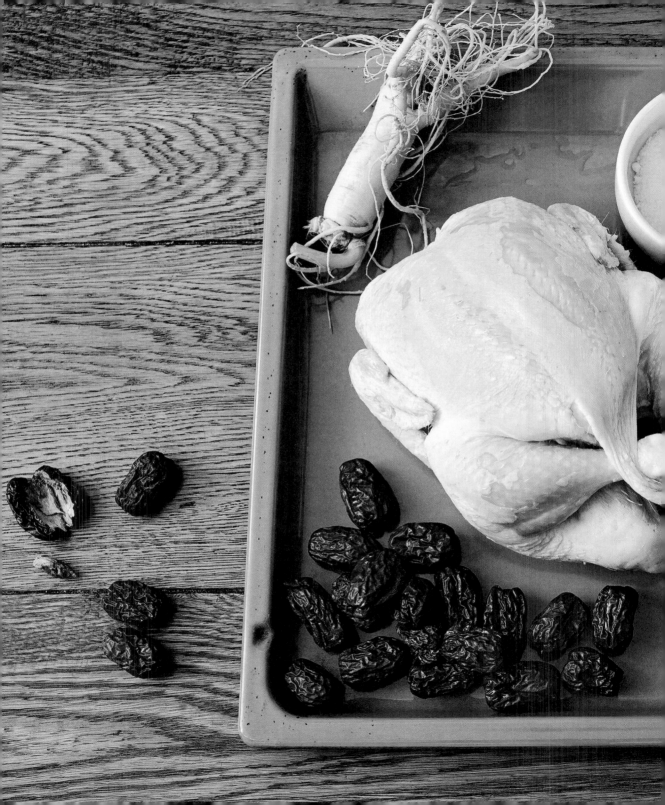

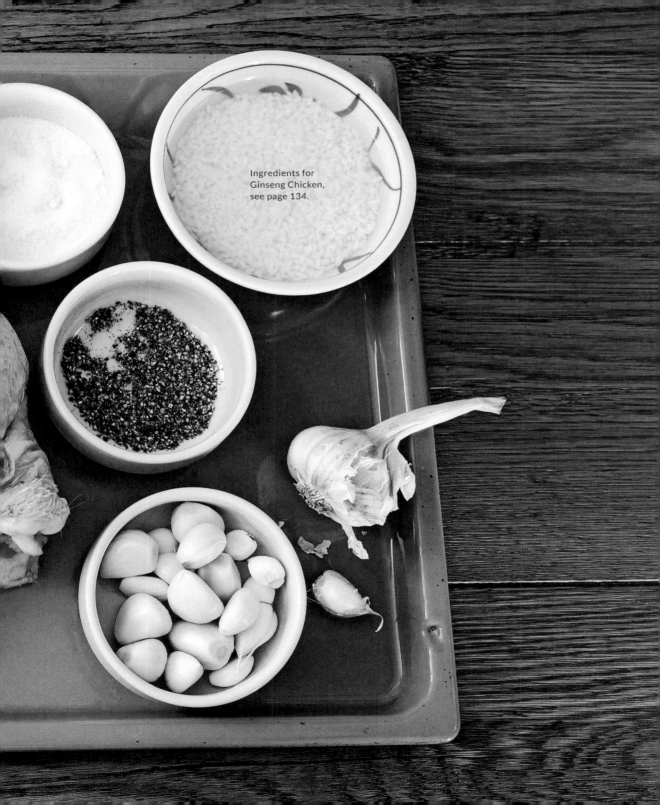

Ingredients for
Ginseng Chicken,
see page 134.

SAMGYETANG

GINSENG CHICKEN

Feeling a bit under the weather? *Samgyetang*, the stew with ginseng, is regarded in Korea as an unrivalled energy boost that makes you strong and warm. There are special *samgyetang* restaurants that serve different variations of the stew – some slightly more expensive ones contain even more healing power in the form of additional wild medicinal plants. Historically, the chicken is cooked in a clay pot with a lid in a traditional clay oven. It can be difficult to source ginseng roots, but you can also use dried ginseng. If so, crush it using a pestle and mortar.

1. Soak the rice for 30 minutes. Drain off the water.
2. Wash the chicken and pat dry. Peel the garlic cloves. Stuff the chicken with the soaked rice, jujube fruits or goji berries, garlic cloves and ginseng roots. Close up the cavity at the tail end of the chicken by making a hole in the skin of each thigh and threading the end of each leg through it, crossing them over (see image on p.132). This should help keep the stuffing inside. Alternatively tie the legs together with string.
3. Place the chicken in a large casserole dish or pan and cover with water. Bring to the boil and leave to simmer covered with a lid for approx. 1½ hours.
4. Mix together the ingredients for the sesame salt on a little plate or in a bowl.
5. Carve and slice up the chicken and eat together with the stuffing and a bowl of boiled rice. Dip the chicken in the sesame salt.

80g/2¾oz/scant ½ cup sticky rice with high gluten content
1 whole chicken, approx. 1.3kg/3lb
1 whole garlic bulb
8 jujube fruits or 50g/1¾oz/heaped ⅓ cup goji berries
Approx. 50g/1¾oz ginseng roots

Sesame salt
4 tbsp sesame oil
1 tbsp salt
1 pinch black pepper

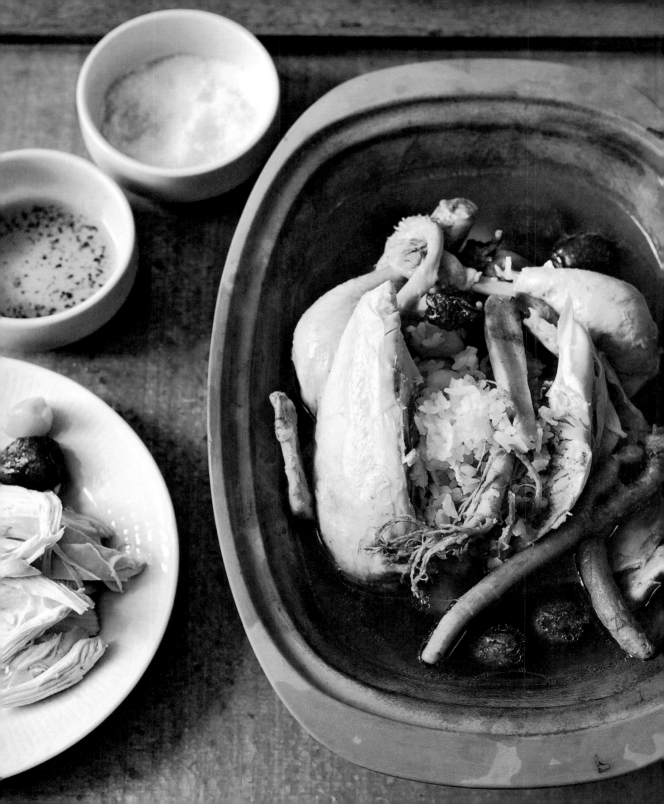

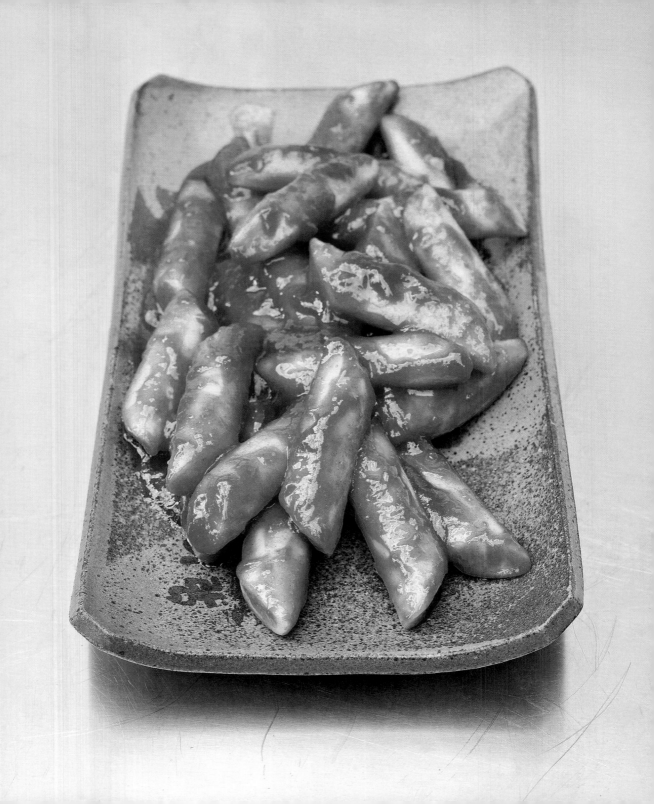

TTEOKBOKKI

FRIED SOFT RICE CAKE IN CHILLI SAUCE

This is an incredibly popular street food in Korea. The most common variety is served with a hot sauce made from *gochujang*. *Tteok* or 'sticky rice' is rice that has been boiled together into a mass. It can be bought in Asian food stores.

'Our grandmother used to make tteokbokki *with sweet soy sauce, sesame oil, some distilled vinegar and shredded carrots and cucumber. And anything our grandmother touched turned magically tasty.'*

1. Heat up *tteok* and water in a frying pan on medium heat.
2. Mix together chilli paste, sugar and sesame oil in a separate bowl and add to the pan once the *tteok* has started to soften. Fry for a few minutes until you get a sticky, fairly thick sauce.
3. Eat the rice cakes as a snack.

1 pack of *tteok*, approx. 500g/1lb 2oz
4 tbsp water
3 tbsp *gochujang*, Korean chilli paste
2 tbsp granulated sugar
1 tbsp sesame oil

OTHER KOREAN DISHES

✓ 깍두기
✓ 열무무김치
✓ 열무 김치
✓ 부추김치

∨ 총각 김치

∨ 배추김치
배추 굴김치 (2/9.)
배추 섞김치 (2/9)

갓절이
오이 김치
호박 김치 (늙은호박, 무청, 배추껍데기)

○ 나박 (양배추) ∨
○ 당근 김치 ∨

동치미
나박김치

백 김치 ✓
꼬들 김치 ?
파 김치
Kålrot 김치

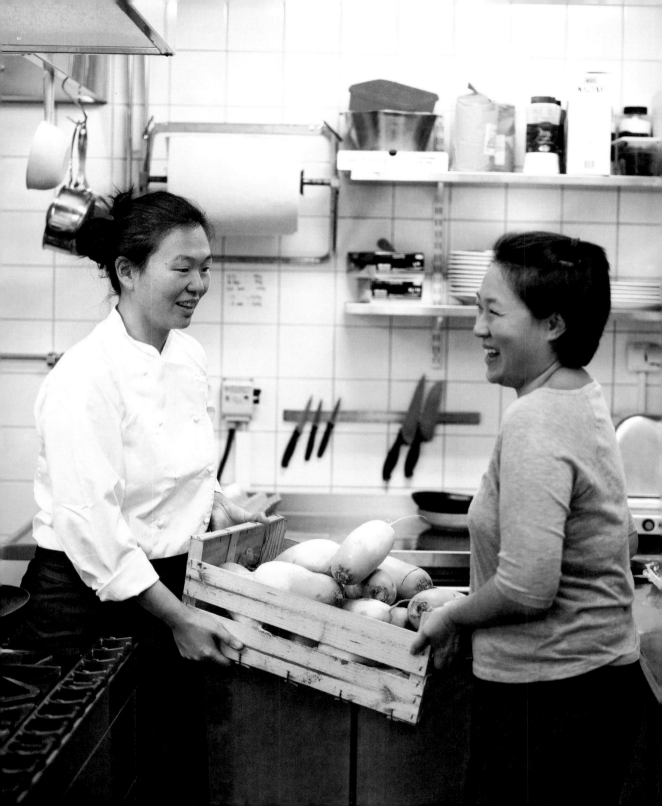

Anju bar snacks
Baechu Chinese leaf/cabbage
Banchan side dishes
Bap cooked rice
Bibimbap mixed rice and meat dish
Bindatteok pancake
Buchu Korean chives
Bul fire
Bulgogi grilled beef
Chunjang black soya bean paste
Daikon white radish, also known as Japanese radish or mooli
Dangmyeon sweet potato flour noodles
Dolsot traditional stone bowl for serving bibimbap or other hot stews
Gim see Kim
Gochu chilli
Gochugaru Korean red chilli powder, available in Asian supermarkets or online by mail order
Gochujang Korean red chilli paste is a traditional Korean condiment used to bring rich spiciness to soups and stews, or add excitement to a bowl of plain rice.
Hobak Korean courgette
Japchae stirfried sweet potato noodles
Jujube red dates
Kim flat dark seaweed sheets, sometimes known as gim, similar to Japanese nori
Kimbap rice and meat snack roll

Kimchi pickled and fermented vegetables
KKaennip see Perilla leaf
Mandu savoury dumplings
Memil myeon buckwheat noodles
Mil myeon wheat noodles
Mul/mul kimchi water/ water kimchi
Myeon cooked noodles
Naengmyeon Korean buckwheat noodles
Namul vegetable side dishes
Oi Korean cucumber
Pajeon pancake
Perilla leaf a member of the mint family, also known as kkaennip and sometimes referred to as sesame leaves, although they are not related to the sesame plant. The leaves are broad and round to spade-like in shape with serrated edges and are aromatic and herbaceous in flavour with nuances of mint, basil and anise.
Soju grain or sweet potato spirit
Tteok rice cakes
Yeolmu baby daikon
Water kimchi a cool refereshing style of kimchi, without chilli, such as Dong Kimchi

INDEX

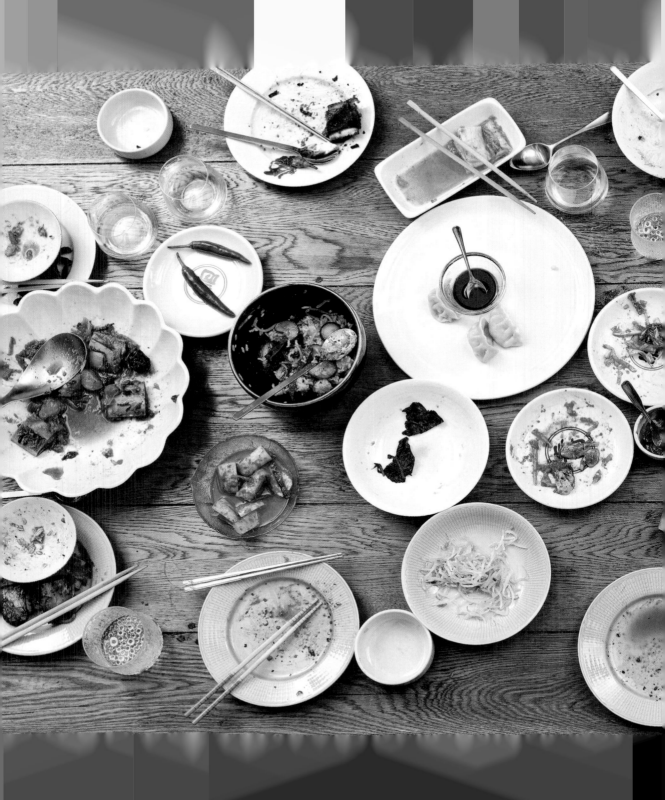

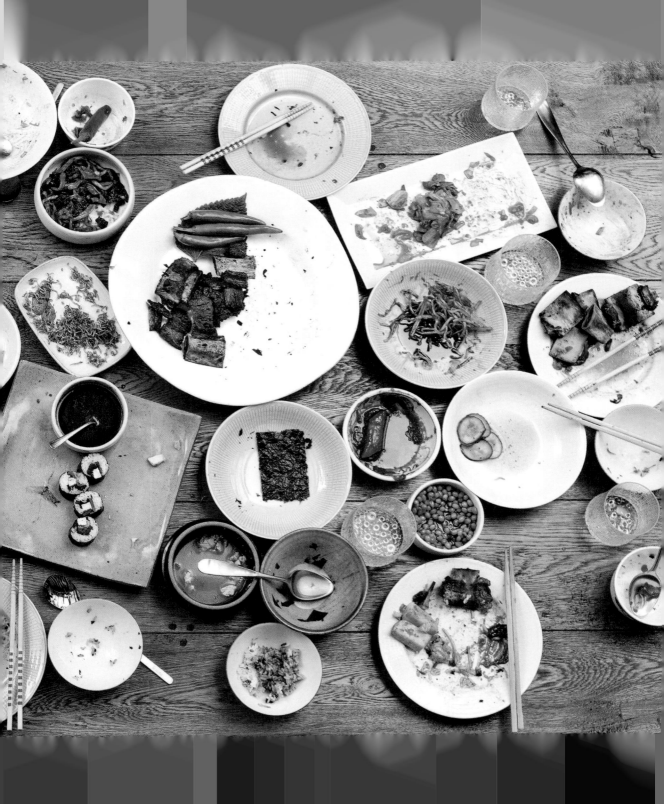

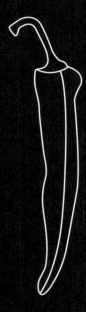

First published in the United Kingdom in 2014 by
Pavilion
1 Gower Street
London WC1E 6HD

This book can be ordered direct from the
publisher at www.pavilionbooks.com

Commisioning editor: Emily Preece-Morrison
Translator: Frida Green

ISBN: 978-1-909815-85-8

A CIP catalogue record for this book is available
from the British Library.

10 9 8 7 6 5 4 3 2

Reproduction by Mission Productions Ltd, Hong Kong
Printed and bound by 1010 Printing International Ltd,
China

First published in Sweden in 2014 as
Kimchi och andra Koreanska Rätter
by Natur & Kultur, Stockholm
www.nok.se

© 2014 Byung-Hi Lim, Byung-Soon Lim
Natur & Kultur, Stockholm
Photography: Anna Kern
Design and Illustrations: Kristin Lidström
Text: Henrik Francke
Editor: Maria Nilsson